To Robert,
Who I loved for who he was.
But he never really understood
that (or he really was not care)

Victoria
september 2015

O'K or Maybe

The Cure Conspiracy:

Medical Myths, Alternative Therapies, and Natural Remedies Even Your Doctor May Not Know

Publisher's Note

The editors of FC&A have taken careful measures to ensure the accuracy and usefulness of the information in this book. While every attempt was made to assure accuracy, some Web sites, addresses, telephone numbers, and other information may have changed since printing.

This book is intended for general information only. It does not constitute medical advice or practice. We cannot guarantee the safety or effectiveness of any treatment or advice mentioned. Readers are urged to consult with their health care professionals.

The publisher and editors disclaim all liability resulting from the use of the information in this book.

"It's in Christ that we find out who we are and what we are living for. Long before we first heard of Christ ... he had his eye on us, had designs on us for glorious living, part of the overall purpose he is working out in everything and everyone."

Ephesians 1:11

Table of contents by remedy

For a list of health conditions, see the *Table of contents by condition* on page vi.

Table of contents by condition

Crack the code on health claims

People just like you spend millions of dollars every year on alternative remedies that don't work in the hope of finding one that does. But fake cures rob you of more than your money — they can also steal your health.

Almost anything goes in the alternative health industry. Companies promise overnight success and miraculous cures with every new supplement, therapy, or wearable device. Some of these remedies may indeed help, but others are just snake oil hawked by slick salesmen.

Treatments that don't work waste your money, and they may keep you from getting real help for health problems. Plus, unproven remedies are often unsafe. Supplements, for instance, can be laced with lead, cause life-threatening side effects, and interact with prescription medications.

It's up to you to sort the good from the bad, the promising cures from the empty promises. Fortunately, this book can help. Here's what it can do for you:

- warn you about the latest fake cures and teach you how to spot phony claims.

- tell you how to safeguard your health when choosing supplements and other alternative therapies.

- help you tap into the healing power of herbs by giving you hard facts on healing herbs that work, hyped-up ones that don't, and which ones to just steer clear of.

- bring you interviews with top experts on new treatments for everything from leg cramps to Alzheimer's disease.

- give you the latest evidence and need-to-know information about dozens of illnesses and remedies.

- explain the science behind each would-be remedy in easy terms you can understand.

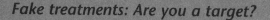

Fake treatments: Are you a target?

Products promising unrealistic, unachievable results tend to target people with chronic or incurable health problems. Often, these victims are desperate for answers because nothing else has helped.

Take extra care investigating alternative therapies, especially if you suffer from one of these illnesses.

- obesity
- arthritis
- memory loss
- Alzheimer's disease
- cancer
- diabetes
- insomnia
- impotence
- heart disease

Spot fake cures and false claims

Hucksters hawk wares they know don't work, and they trade on your hope in the bargain. Don't be fooled by false promises. Learn to see through their lies so you can look for treatments that do help.

Remember, if something sounds too good to be true, it probably is. Beware of any product that:

- makes unrealistic claims to treat a wide variety of illnesses, such as "benefits arthritis, heart disease, ulcers, memory loss, and more!"

- suggests it cures or treats serious illnesses, especially those your doctor says don't have a cure

- uses sensational words like "miraculous cure," "revolutionary innovation," "scientific breakthrough," or "secret ingredient"

- uses impressive scientific-sounding words, such as "thermogenesis"

- presents personal testimonials from unnamed people or doctors who claim unbelievable results
- asks for advance payment
- warns you that supplies are limited or pressures you to decide on the spot
- promises no-risk, money-back guarantees
- doesn't list the company's name, address, and phone number in the ad or on the Web site
- claims that scientists and other medical professionals are trying to hide the miracle-product or don't want you to learn about it

'Natural' does not mean safe

Why put harsh drugs in your body when you have so many safe, natural, gentle options, like herbs and other supplements?

Unfortunately, 'natural' products are not always harmless and wholesome. It's the biggest lie in health care. Sure, many supplements have real benefits, but not everything for sale is safe.

The Food and Drug Administration (FDA) does not regulate the safety or quality of dietary supplements the way it does drugs. Here are some key ways supplements differ from prescription and over-the-counter medications.

- New supplements do not have to be approved for sale by the FDA or any government agency.
- Supplement makers do not have to prove their products are safe or effective before selling them.
- Nor do they have to report complaints they receive about side effects and serious health problems caused by a supplement.

- The government does not require warning labels on potentially dangerous supplements the way it does on medications.

- Supplement manufacturers do not have to regulate the quality of their products.

- They can make claims about a supplement's healing powers without solid scientific evidence to back them.

Supplement manufacturers are expected to regulate themselves, a little like asking the fox to guard the hen house. That could leave you with a few unpleasant surprises.

Side effects can be serious. Herbs, extracts, and other supplements have side effects, too, just like medications. Your

Coral calcium cures cancer?

Fiction: Coral calcium from Okinawa, Japan, can cure over 200 illnesses, including heart disease, Alzheimer's, and cancer.

Fact: The only thing these supplements are sure to do is put a dent in your wallet.

Calcium helps prevent osteoporosis, and it may help lower blood pressure and reduce your risk of colorectal cancer. But coral calcium works no better than other calcium supplements, and it has never been proven to cure anything.

Supplement makers claim that Okinawans live longer, healthier lives because they consume coral calcium. Actually, it's largely due to their active lifestyle and diet of vegetables, fish, and grains.

Promoters also claim your body absorbs 100 percent of the calcium from coral calcium, compared to 1 percent from other supplements. In truth, your body only absorbs 25 to 35 percent of the calcium in any supplement, including coral calcium.

The Federal Trade Commission has charged the people marketing this product with making unsubstantiated claims. Think twice before you buy their sales pitch.

doctor helps monitor your reactions to prescription drugs, but with supplements, you're often on your own. You may not notice a problem until it's too late.

- Comfrey, an herb long used as a poultice for achy joints and bruises, may lead to cancer and contains alkaloids, which can cause serious liver damage.

- Kava kava, a popular herb to relieve anxiety, stress, and insomnia, can also cause liver failure. Several countries have banned it, but it is still sold in the United States.

- Large doses of certain vitamins and minerals can harm you, too. High doses of vitamin A over long periods reduces bone density and may lead to liver damage and birth defects.

Toxins taint. You could also get more than you bargained for, including contaminants like lead. A respected independent lab recently found dangerous amounts of lead in both a brand of coral calcium and a memory enhancer made with huperzine A.

Drugs don't mix. Seemingly harmless supplements may interact with medications. St. John's Wort, for instance, can react with blood-thinners, antidepressants, and transplant drugs. Ginkgo biloba, a relatively safe herb, can trigger excessive bleeding if taken with aspirin, heparin, warfarin, or other blood-thinning medications.

Safety comes second. Stores and Web sites can legally sell supplements known to cause serious health problems, like those containing kava kava. What's worse, you may never even realize a product is dangerous since warning labels are voluntary, not required. And while drugs come with product information explaining their risks, supplements often don't, even though they pose similar hazards.

Labels lie. You never really know what you're getting because no one regulates quality. Many supplements don't even contain the ingredients they claim.

Lose weight fast?

Ephedra, or Ma Huang, is an herbal stimulant once used widely in diet pills and weight loss supplements. Unfortunately, promoters exaggerated its benefits, and for years, they covered up its life-threatening side effects.

Ephedra seems to raise your blood pressure and may cause irregular heartbeats, seizures, heart attacks, and strokes. Evidence links it to 155 deaths.

The Food and Drug Administration spent seven years collecting enough evidence to ban the herb from dietary supplements. Finally, in February 2004, it succeeded.

Three other "natural" weight loss products pose similar risks.

- Fen-phen has been linked to heart damage and removed from the market.
- Phenylpropanolamine (PPA) causes your blood pressure to sky-rocket.
- Bitter orange, or *Citrus aurantium*, works like ephedra. It may also raise your blood pressure and cause heart problems.

- In recent lab tests, one-third of probiotic supplements had less than 1 percent of the live bacteria promised on their labels.

- The same goes for ginkgo supplements. Less than one-fourth of them met quality standards in independent lab tests in 2003.

- More than half of cholesterol-lowering products, including guggelsterone, failed lab tests because either they did not contain the ingredients they claimed or they did not break down inside the body.

Sharpen your supplement savvy

Your best defense against unsafe supplements and phony therapies is to be a smart consumer. Learn the facts backing a product or treatment, get trustworthy advice, and complain if you think you've been taken for a ride.

Scope out supplements. You can't always count on a supplement's label to tell you what it contains. The independent laboratory ConsumerLab.com has made a name for itself testing health and nutrition products for quality and safety. They publish their results on their Web site, *www.ConsumerLab.com*.

Here you can find out which supplement brands had the right amount of active ingredients, which did not, and which posed health hazards. You can read partial results from their tests for free, but to see the full reports, you must subscribe to their service the way you would a magazine.

Read up on recalls. The Food and Drug Administration (FDA) issues warnings about supplements as soon as they learn of potential dangers. Stay up to date by visiting their Web site at *www.cfsan.fda.gov* and clicking on "Dietary Supplements," or call the FDA's toll-free information line 1-888-463-6332.

ConsumerLab.com also publishes recalls, warnings, and other alerts on their Web site. You can read the latest alert for free, but you must subscribe to their service to see old ones.

Ask your doctor. Considering a supplement or alternative therapy? Run it past your doctor. She can warn you about the dangers, help

> Sometimes the FDA and Federal Trade Commission (FTC) take legal action against sellers, especially those who lie about the healing powers or safety of their product. Find out who's guilty at *www.ftc.gov* or *www.fda.gov/oc/enforcement.html*.

you watch for side effects, and avoid prescribing medicine that could interact with your supplements.

Make your complaint heard. The FDA collects complaints about supplement side effects and uses them to build a case against dangerous products. You or your doctor should report supplement-related side effects to the FDA by calling 1-800-332-1088 or filling out a form online at *www.fda.gov/medwatch*.

Do your own research. Too often, sellers exaggerate the benefits of their products. Find out for yourself what hard science says about an alternative treatment. Look for these reliable books at your local library.

- *Tyler's Honest Herbal* by Steven Foster and Varro Tyler
- *Botanical Medicines* by Dennis J. McKenna, Kenneth Jones, and Kerry Hughes

Boost brainpower with Focus Factor?

Focus Factor claims to provide nutritional support for your underfed brain. It promises to improve your memory, mental clarity, and concentration; enable you to recall numbers, facts, and names; increase your energy; fight fatigue; relieve stress, irritability, and mood swings — and all in as few as one to 10 days.

The Federal Trade Commission (FTC) says otherwise. It has fined the promoters of Focus Factor more than $1 million dollars for making unsubstantiated claims. The FTC says the sellers of this 'hot' supplement do not have scientific evidence to back their claims and that they paid people to endorse their product and give testimonials.

A mere month's supply costs $50 or more, but experts say don't waste your money. Instead, discuss symptoms like memory loss with your doctor. He can tell if they are linked to a nutritional deficiency and offer proven treatments.

- *Alternative Medicine: The Definitive Guide*, 2nd edition, by Burton Goldberg, John W. Anderson, and Larry Trivieri

A few Web sites offer easy-to-read, unbiased information about herbs, nutrition, and alternative treatments. For instance, the Office of Dietary Supplements, a department of the National Institutes of Health (NIH), provides information about supplement safety and side effects. Visit their Web site at *http://dietary-supplements.info.nih.gov* and click on "Health Information." Check out these resources for additional advice.

- National Center for Complementary and Alternative Medicine at *www.nccam.nih.gov*

- MayoClinic.com at *www.mayoclinic.com*

Next, you'll learn about the research behind discoveries and how to make sense of new findings yourself.

Secrets to testing new treatments

Scientists often start off with an idea about what causes a disease or how a treatment might help. But no matter how much sense a theory makes, it isn't truth until researchers test it.

It's not enough for someone to swear an herb or magnetic bracelet will cure your arthritis. You need to see solid evidence supporting those claims — not just opinions or testimonials, but medical trials in real people that prove they do.

That's one reason health experts are skeptical of many supplements and alternative remedies. Often, no studies have proven they really

Only about five out of 5,000 chemical compounds tested in the lab eventually get tested in humans, and only one of those five may be safe and effective enough to become a drug available at your pharmacy.

work, or in what dosages and at what risks. Only careful research can do that.

Just consider prescription medications. The Food and Drug Administration (FDA) says drug companies spend, on average, eight-and-a-half years developing and testing a new medication before it gains FDA approval. Here's a snapshot of what happens.

- A drug company decides to develop a new treatment for an illness.

- Researchers spend years, even decades, studying the processes and chemicals in the body that lead to the health problem.

- Once they understand how the illness happens, they do test tube experiments to find a chemical compound — a future drug — that stops the disease from developing. They may try thousands of substances to find a few that work.

- Experts figure out how each successful compound stops the disease. Then they adjust the chemical makeup of each substance to make it more effective.

- Next, they test these potential drugs in two or more types of animals to learn how well each works, how much gets absorbed into the bloodstream, the safety of different doses, and possible side effects.

- Depending on animal results, experts may go back and alter a drug's chemistry to make it even more effective. This may take more test tube experiments, and then more animal tests.

- The FDA reviews animal results to decide if a drug is safe enough to test in people.

- A panel of scientists, ethicists, and others look over the plans for human trials to make sure they are safe and ethical.

- If so, drug companies begin clinical trials in small groups of healthy people to discover the most common side effects of each drug and how high a dose people can safely tolerate. These studies last several months.

- If all goes well, researchers begin studies in people who have the illness the drug was made to treat to find out if it helps. This could take several months to two years.

- Next, they test the medication in an even larger group of people. This could last one to four years.

- If the drug works safely in all of these studies, the drug company asks the FDA for approval to sell it.

- The FDA looks at the clinical trial results to decide if the benefits of the drug outweigh its risks and side effects. If so, the FDA may approve it.

Learn the basics of health research

Everything doctors know about your health comes from research, research, and more research. Doing the research might be difficult, but reading about it doesn't have to be.

Decoding science-speak is easy once you know a few simple terms. Basically, scientists use five types of studies to unravel medical mysteries. Each has strengths and weaknesses, and it generally takes all of them to solve the riddle of a disease.

Lab test. Big discoveries start out small, often in a test tube or Petri dish. Here, lab researchers study chemical compounds, trying to understand how they affect cells and other tiny organisms, like bacteria and viruses. In fact, that's how researchers discovered penicillin — through lab tests.

These experiments help scientists figure out how drugs and the body work. But what happens in a test tube is not necessarily what will happen in your body. Lab findings are just the beginning, and they don't translate directly to people. Researchers need to do animal and human tests to confirm their lab results.

Cough remedy cures fibromyalgia?

Rumors that guaifenesin, an ingredient in cough syrup that loosens mucus, treats fibromyalgia have persisted for years, despite all evidence to the contrary.

In theory, it might work. Supporters believe calcium phosphate builds up in the muscles and tendons of some people, causing fibromyalgia. They say guaifenesin helps your kidneys get rid of uric acid, which in turn flushes out the excess calcium phosphate and eventually cures the disease.

Researchers at Oregon Health Sciences University conducted a year-long randomized, double-blinded, placebo-controlled clinical trial to see if it worked. People with fibromyalgia taking 600 milligrams of guaifenesin twice a day showed no improvement in strength, distance walked without pain, quality of life, or number and size of tender points compared to placebo. Nor did they excrete more uric acid or calcium phosphate.

While the guaifenesin theory sounds believable, good research reveals it doesn't hold up. New studies suggest this disease actually stems from a problem in the central nervous system, not the muscles.

Animal test. Animal research helps scientists understand what effect drugs, nutrients, and other substances might have in people.

The important thing for you to remember — the results of animal studies don't apply directly to people, either. Researchers usually give animals much higher dosages of a substance than most humans would ever receive, and animals sometimes react differently to compounds than humans do. So just because animal studies show a treatment doesn't work, or that a substance causes cancer, scientists don't know for sure until they study people.

Epidemiologic study. Epidemiologists observe people to find links between health problems and diet, living habits, or other factors. Say, for instance, experts track the eating and living habits of 5,000 people in Chicago for 10 years. At the end, they may notice that people taking cholesterol-lowering statin drugs did not develop Alzheimer's disease as often as other people. In fact, that's exactly how researchers discovered statin drugs may prevent Alzheimer's.

Epidemiologic research can suggest links, but it cannot prove cause and effect. "Epidemiologic studies don't show whether something works or not. They show an association," says Dr. Allan Levey, professor and chairman of the Department of Neurology at Emory University and director of the Emory Alzheimer's Disease Center.

"For instance, epidemiologic studies have suggested very good evidence that people who take statins have a lower risk of Alzheimer's disease," he explains. "Now what these types of studies don't tell you is whether the statin is responsible for reducing that risk. For example, the same people who take statins might also be more educated, eat a better diet, exercise more, smoke less, or have lower blood pressure." These are all factors that lower people's risk of Alzheimer's disease.

Epidemiologic research can point to clues, but it can't offer final answers. "That's where clinical trials are important," Levey says. Only they can prove which treatments work and which don't.

Clinical trial. In this type of study, scientists test people to confirm or expand on the results of lab, animal, and epidemiologic studies. Often, researchers give them a drug, supplement, or other therapy to see if it really does treat or prevent a certain disease.

A certain percentage of people feel better when they start taking medicine, even if that medication is fake. This improvement is called the placebo effect, and it can throw off the results of clinical trials. Placebo-controlling counteracts the placebo effect to keep it from skewing the study's results.

Good clinical trials are essential to proving whether a remedy works. The better structured a trial, the more reliable its results. The best clinical studies have these three traits.

- **Randomized.** Researchers recruit people then randomly assign each one to either the control or test group. The test group gets the new treatment, while the control group does not. This random assignment keeps researchers from subconsciously biasing the groups, for instance, by putting the healthiest people in the test group so the new treatment appears to work.

- **Placebo-controlled.** The control group usually receives a placebo, a fake pill such as a sugar pill, which looks exactly like the real drug. This way, no one knows if they are receiving the treatment or not. If the new treatment does not work, researchers may say the therapy worked no better than placebo.

- **Double-blinded.** This means neither the people in the experiment nor the researchers themselves know who is getting the real medicine and who is getting the placebo. It's one more way to control researcher bias and the placebo effect, so it makes the results more accurate.

The best clinical trials meet the "gold standard" — they are randomized, double-blinded, and placebo-controlled. Scientists cannot design every trial like this. For instance, you can't double-blind a garlic study — but they try.

Meta-analysis. Researchers use a statistical report, a meta-analysis, to pool the results of many separate studies on a treatment. Scientists often do a meta-analysis when trials don't offer a clear answer about whether a remedy works.

For example, some clinical trials on St. Johns Wort for depression show the herb helps, while others show it doesn't. To conduct a meta-analysis, experts would collect all the results from past trials of St. Johns Wort for depression, then analyze them to see how effective it is overall.

These reports aren't perfect, and, once again, they aren't a final say. But done well, they are a good tool for finding out how well a treatment works.

Keep research in perspective

You have every right to be skeptical about new health recommendations. Every day, experts seem to change their minds about what you should eat, drink, and do to stay healthy, and new research constantly contradicts old findings.

Trying to keep up with every new discovery can drive you crazy. The secret to saving your sanity — keep new research in perspective, and wait before you make drastic changes or stock up on the latest super supplement.

Take new studies with a grain of salt. Carrots cure cancer! The media likes to portray new research as if it offers the final, revolutionary answer to all your problems. But rarely does one piece of research solve anything.

Think of an illness, like colon cancer, as a puzzle. Each study is another piece. When researchers finish a trial, they try to figure out how their piece — their findings — fit into the larger puzzle. Sometimes they put together lots of pieces with one study, but more often it takes many studies to connect a few pieces.

Get a look at the big picture. You can't tell what a puzzle picture looks like just from one piece — and no study can stand on its own. Always consider it in light of the pieces around it. Any good news report should put the latest findings in perspective, telling you what past research said about a treatment or illness, and how the new evidence fits in.

Wait for more proof. You don't have to follow the advice of every new finding. In fact, you probably shouldn't if it goes against all the previous health advice you heard. Any new study that contradicts past research will require much more testing before scientists adopt it as truth. Discuss the results with your doctor before making any drastic changes in your diet, lifestyle, or medication.

Sniff out suspect studies

Even if the researchers get it right, studies can still go wrong down the line. Pitfalls in the publishing or reporting of health information can lead you and even experts to the wrong conclusions. Beware of these potential flaws and factor them into how much faith you put in new findings.

Funding sources. Studies are expensive to conduct, and all that money has to come from somewhere. The government and many independent agencies award grants for research, but pharmaceutical, supplement, and other industries also fund studies.

Once scientists complete their testing, they submit their results to medical journals. When they do, they are also supposed to disclose who gave them money for their research, and if they have any affiliation with a health company, like a drug manufacturer.

Industry funding doesn't necessarily make a study biased, but some experts think the results are more accurate and objective if a third party, like the government, funded it instead. Some evidence agrees. For instance, industry-funded trials are more likely to show a new treatment, such as a drug, works than are trials funded by independent groups, like the government.

Find out who funded the study when you hear evidence trumpeting a new therapy. If the health industry had a hand in it, look at other studies on the same topic to see what they say.

Publication bias. Studies showing positive results are more likely to get published, and get published faster, than those showing a treatment doesn't work or is actually harmful. That means you and your doctor are more likely to hear about studies that support a treatment.

This trend worries scientists because it doesn't tell them the whole story about new therapies, like drugs. For example, the government has sued one drug company for hiding studies that show its drug does not work in a certain group of people and that it can cause severe, life-threatening side effects.

Researchers doing a meta-analysis check for publication bias to keep it from skewing their results. You can do your own check by discussing treatments you want to try, including alternative therapies, with a doctor you trust.

Sensational reporting. Medical journals and pharmaceutical companies aren't the only ones to blame for bias. News reporters and their editors may play an even bigger part in what health breakthroughs you hear about and the important details you don't.

Writers and reporters are short on time and space, under pressure to make tough decisions about which details you need and which you can do without. To get your attention, they sometimes sacrifice important but boring study specifics for attention-grabbing headlines and impressive numbers.

Be skeptical of the hype surrounding any supposed health "breakthrough." Rarely do scientists make a major, surprising advancement. More often, science moves forward at a slow but steady pace. Pay close attention to the study details the media reports and judge for yourself how much stock to put in them based on your newfound knowledge of health research.

Top 7 details to look for in research

Too often, the media use hyped-up headlines to grab your attention. But what does a study really say?

Any good health article or news report should tell you some basic information about the research that led to a new finding. Look for these details when deciding how much faith you should put in the results.

- Was the study done in test tubes, animals, or people? Lab and animal results don't always apply well to people.

- If it was a human study, was it a clinical trial or epidemiologic study? Remember, only clinical trials can prove cause and effect.

- If it was a clinical trial, did it meet the gold standard?

- How many people did researchers study and for how long? Generally, the more people a study includes and the longer it lasts, the more reliable its results.

- How does the new evidence fit in with old research? A good reporter will put the findings in perspective.

- Was the study funded by a commercial industry, such as a supplement or drug company, or by a nonbiased group, like the National Institutes of Health?

- Did the journalist present a balanced view of the topic, with the strengths and weaknesses of the study or interviews with experts on both sides of a controversial issue?

Quick tips for reading this book

Wondering if aspirin really does prevent Alzheimer's? And what's the story behind magnetic bracelets? This book will explain what works and what doesn't with simple yet in-depth answers and real advice you can trust. Each chapter in this amazing book:

- delivers the latest buzz about a popular "cure"

- explains in clear, simple terms what the treatment entails and how experts think it works — or doesn't

- gives you the scoop on the research behind a remedy and what the results mean for you

- offers practical advice, including warnings, side effects, and expert tips for making the most of each remedy

You'll learn if garlic cures colds, how chocolate could conquer heart disease, whether guggul really lowers cholesterol, and how tomatoes could crush both cancer and osteoporosis, among many other remedies on the cutting edge of today's science.

Each chapter covers a different remedy. You can head straight to the remedy you want to read about, or check the index for a particular health problem and the treatments that could help.

Best of all, each remedy is rated from no star to three stars to help you determine how trustworthy the treatment is.

 No star — Steer clear. The remedy is either totally bogus or has virtually no solid evidence to back it.

 One star — Consider with caution. Early research suggests the treatment might work, but experts need to study it more before they can recommend it. Some one-star remedies may help a few people but not everyone.

Two stars — The future looks bright. Good scientific evidence suggests this remedy works, and some doctors recommend it. But researchers still have reservations about how safe or effective it is, and they need to study it more.

Three stars — All systems go. This remedy is an established treatment. It has gone through a long, thorough research process, and health experts feel confident prescribing it.

Right now, no miracle remedy will cure you of arthritis, guarantee you'll never get heart disease, or completely guard you against Alzheimer's and other serious conditions. However, a number of remedies can lower your risk of getting a certain disease or improve your quality of life if you already have it. Don't lose hope. Get started on the road to healing now.

ACE inhibitors for high blood pressure

★★★

Wonder drug for blood vessels

ACE inhibitors have been around since the 1980s. Yet, little was known about how they work until recently. New research is shedding light on how these remarkable drugs do their job. Amazingly, ACE (angiotensin-converting enzyme) inhibitors don't just reduce blood pressure. They also improve the health of your arteries.

How it works

ACE inhibitors are prescription drugs that block angiotensin II, a powerful enzyme that narrows blood vessels. They help blood vessel walls relax, which lowers your blood pressure and allows more blood and oxygen to reach your heart. But there's more.

While it's normal for blood vessel cells to die, high blood pressure causes the cells to die faster than they can be replaced by new cells — from 1.3 percent every 30 minutes in a healthy person to 7.8 percent every 30 minutes in someone who has high blood pressure. This increase results in scarring and plaque build-up in the arteries. That's where ACE inhibitors come in.

ACE inhibitors to the rescue

Two important studies have confirmed the wonder drug status of ACE inhibitors. The most recent, nicknamed EUROPA, involved 20,000 participants and focused on the ACE inhibitor perindopril's ability to prevent heart attacks, as well as reduce plaque buildup.

The other, HOPE, is a five-year study that followed 9,000 people taking ramipril, another ACE inhibitor. All 9,000 study

> ## *Know your blood pressure numbers*
>
> If your blood pressure reading is 120/80, you may think you have nothing to worry about. In reality, you are considered prehypertensive and at risk for developing full-blown hypertension, or high blood pressure.
>
> In 2003, the National Heart, Lung, and Blood Institute released guidelines based on new knowledge that damage to arteries begins at fairly low blood-pressure levels — levels once considered normal, even good.
>
> It's important to know your numbers and lower your blood pressure if needed. According to the Centers for Disease Control, taking this precaution could cut your chances of suffering heart disease or stroke by 33 to 50 percent.
>
> Here's what you need to remember.
> - "Normal" is less than 120 over less than 80 mm Hg.
> - "Prehypertension" is 120-139 over 80-89 mm Hg.
> - "Stage 1 hypertension" is 140-159 over 90-99 mm Hg.
> - "Stage 2 hypertension" means at or greater than 160 over at or greater than 100 mm Hg.

participants had heart disease, diabetes, or had suffered a stroke. They also had at least one other risk factor for heart disease, like high blood pressure, high cholesterol levels, or smoking.

Both studies demonstrated the remarkable ability of ACE inhibitors to do their job — and more. HOPE researchers found that the ACE inhibitor they studied not only lowered blood pressure, it reduced the risk of heart attack and diabetes.

Surprisingly, the people who took it were 30 percent less likely to develop diabetes and far less likely to have heart attacks — 150 fewer for every 1,000 people treated over a four-year period.

In a spinoff of the EUROPA study, researchers discovered something interesting. Participants with heart disease who took an ACE inhibitor saw the death rate of cells lining their arteries plummet from 7.3 percent to 4.7 percent at the end of the study. That translates to a major improvement in the health of artery walls, making them more resistant to plaque.

ACE inhibitors are well tolerated and have no ill effects on sexual desire or performance. Some users actually report they improve their mood. What's more, they're also being prescribed for diabetes-related kidney problems.

And the future looks very promising — scientists say the next generation of ACE inhibitors will be even more effective.

A few things to consider

Store your ACE inhibitors away from direct light and heat. And keep them away from damp places, like kitchen sinks and bathrooms.

Herbs that boost blood pressure		
Herb	**Scientific name**	**Use**
Cacao	*Theobroma cacao*	Stimulant
Coffee	*Coffea arabica*	Stimulant
Ephedra (Ma huang)	*Ephedra*	Anti-asthmatic, nasal decongestant
Kola	*Cola nitida*	Stimulant
Licorice	*Glycyrrhiza glabra*	Treats coughs and colds
Mistletoe, American	*Phoradendron leucarpum*	Increases blood pressure
Rosemary	*Rosmarinus officinalis*	Stimulant
Tea	*Camellia sinensis*	Stimulant

> It's possible to have a severe reaction to ACE inhibitors even several years after beginning treatment. If you take these medications to regulate your blood pressure, make sure you report any strange reactions — even a mild one, such as tongue swelling that goes away on its own — to your doctor immediately.

If you are taking ACE inhibitors to control high blood pressure, don't use over-the-counter drugs for appetite control, colds, or congestion without first checking with your doctor. Many remedies for these ailments tend to raise blood pressure.

Two infrequent side effects of ACE inhibitors are headaches and dry cough. Usually, the headaches can be tamed with cold packs, a hot shower, controlled breathing, or regular exercise.

As with all prescription drugs, follow your doctor's and pharmacist's instructions carefully.

Acupuncture for osteoarthritis pain

Needles work to block the ache

You would be surprised at the amazing things you can do to help your body heal, such as easing arthritis pain with acupuncture. More than 15 million Americans have tried this ancient Chinese practice to relieve pain.

Nearly everyone over age 70 has some symptoms of osteoarthritis, which is caused by wear and tear on the cartilage in your joints. There is no known cure for osteoarthritis. The best you can do is to slow down the deterioration and manage the pain.

How it works

An acupuncturist sticks several very fine needles — about a dozen for osteoarthritis — into various parts of the body for about 20 minutes. After the needles are removed, many people experience less arthritis pain. Why this works is not exactly clear.

Traditional Chinese acupuncturists insert the needles at specific points related to your condition, according to traditional Chinese medicine (TCM). They believe this regulates the flow of energy, or qi, through your body.

The Western medical community still doesn't understand TCM very well. Medical acupuncturists point out that acupuncture sites contain many nerve endings that stimulate the brain to release natural pain-blocking chemicals called endorphins into your body.

"Regardless of whether you call it qi or endorphins, something's happening," says Dr. Joanne Borg-Stein. She's a specialist in musculoskeletal medicine and in charge of physical medicine and rehabilitation at Newton-Wellesley Hospital, a teaching site for the Harvard Medical School. She's also a medical acupuncturist.

The Harvard physical medicine and rehabilitation faculty uses acupuncture routinely, Borg-Stein says. They have been successful in using acupuncture along with more traditional treatments to make arthritis sufferers better — particularly those with significant or severe osteoarthritis of the knees, hips, spine, or shoulder.

> "When you have a new joint complaint, have at least a one-time medical assessment and some X-rays to make sure it's not something more life-threatening than arthritis," advises Dr. Joanne Borg-Stein.

"We don't change the X-ray pictures," she cautions, "so it is very likely that the symptoms are managed rather than cured. I can treat people for years and keep them very functional."

A good backup treatment

Most experts and studies suggest using acupuncture as an additional treatment if other things aren't working very well. Dr. Borg-Stein agrees.

"If simple treatments, such as weight loss, exercise, judicious use of Tylenol or anti-inflammatory medication, don't allow a patient to be comfortable and function, then they certainly should try acupuncture," she says. Research on how good acupuncture is for osteoarthritis doesn't give very clear answers. Most studies agree that it helps, but it probably shouldn't be used as a first-line treatment. Many experts say it's a good second or third choice and is helpful when used in addition to other treatments.

You should see improvement within your first six to 10 visits to an acupuncturist. If you don't feel better, it might not be a

---

Acupuncture relief without needles

Consider acupressure if you like the idea of acupuncture, but can't stand the thought of someone sticking needles in your body.

Acupressure stimulates the same points as acupuncture but doesn't use needles or break the skin. There are different methods, like focusing on pressure points or using stroking and rubbing motions. The practitioner may use his fingers, whole hand, elbow, or feet, as well as special tools like rollers or balls.

You can even learn to do it yourself. Read up on acupressure at your library, or attend a workshop. One of the basic pain relief spots is in the webbing between your thumb and forefinger. Find a tender spot near the base of your index finger bone with your opposite thumb. Hold it for several seconds to relieve arthritis aches in your hands, arms, neck, or shoulders.

good solution for you. Supplementary treatments every six weeks or two months might be necessary to control pain.

Find a trained therapist

It's a challenge to find a legitimate acupuncturist because there are so many types and theories of acupuncture. Every state has different licensing requirements, and some don't have any at all. Just make sure the acupuncturist you choose is formally trained and has actual experience.

For more information, contact the American Academy of Medical Acupuncture at 800-521-2262 or *www.medicalacupuncture.org* and the National Certification Commission for Acupuncture and Oriental Medicine at 703-548-9004 or *www.nccaom.org*.

The U.S. Food and Drug Administration regulates acupuncture needles. They must be sterile, labeled for single-use only, and used exclusively by state-qualified practitioners. Make sure your acupuncturist uses approved needles.

The cost of acupuncture may be a drawback. Some insurers, including Medicare, won't pay for it. Treatments prescribed or administered by medical doctors are more likely to be covered. Check the requirements of your plan.

Air purifiers for allergies

Gain ground against airborne allergens

Allergens cause allergy sufferers to sneeze, wheeze, and cough. They lurk everywhere — on your pets, in your carpet, bedding, and upholstered furniture, and most importantly, in the air you breathe.

A good air filtering system won't remove them all, but it can be an important member of your anti-allergen team.

How it works

Common airborne allergy triggers include dust, pet allergens, pollen, mold, and tobacco smoke. Of course, not all allergens are airborne. If they're "land-based," air filters won't catch them. But a good filtration system can do a decent job of improving the quality of indoor air.

Air cleaning systems include single-room or area appliances, install-it-yourself central air system filters, and professionally installed "electrostatic precipitators" that work with your central air system. These systems filter airborne particles, capture allergens "electrostatically," or both.

Ordinary filters capture particles that are drawn through the return-air duct. Electrostatic precipitators, on the other hand, are like electrically charged dirt collectors. They attract and capture charged allergen particles with their own opposite electrical charge.

Allergy-related illnesses	Doctor visits in the United States for one year
Allergic rhinitis (allergies and hay fever)	14,101,000
Chronic sinusitis	14,197,000
Asthma	12,692,000

Filter through the research

A study reported in the *Journal of Allergy and Clinical Immunology* looked at the effectiveness of single-room air purifiers in the bedooms and living rooms of asthma patients who had indoor cats and dogs. It found that air cleaners reduced the levels of airborne pet allergens. When used along with other anti-allergen measures, the air cleaners helped asthma patients who wanted to keep their pets.

They could not determine the real effectiveness of air cleaners, though, because they only removed airborne allergens, not those that live in carpet, bedding, and upholstery. Air cleaners can't do it alone.

> To clear your sinuses, dissolve a half teaspoon of salt in a cup of warm water. With a bulb syringe, flush your nose with the mixture.

Another study looked at the results of 10 trials dealing with home air filtering systems and their impact on people with asthma and allergies. It concluded that using air filters, especially HEPA (high-efficiency particulate arresting) filters, results in fewer allergy symptoms and fewer sleep disturbances. But they don't influence how much medication allergy sufferers must use to control their symptoms.

Finally, the Environmental Protection Agency, the government's watchdog for air quality, believes air cleaners may be useful. It warns, however, that air cleaners alone can't assure good air quality, especially if your home has unchecked sources of airborne grime and poor ventilation.

Clear the air of allergens

Whether you use an air purifier or not, you can take these simple steps to cleaner, allergen-free indoor air.

- Ask your doctor to determine which allergens trigger your allergies. Your triggers may all live in the carpet rather than the air, so an air purifier could be an ineffective investment.

- See if simply upgrading your furnace filter or replacing it more often will do the trick.

- Since airborne mold is often the result of moisture, make sure you've fixed all your leaks, or install a dehumidifier. Attack the mold problem at its source.

- Make sure dirty attic or basement air isn't circulating through your house because of leaky seals around attic and basement doors. Those parts of your house can provide a steady supply of dust and other allergens.

To find an effective air-cleaning appliance or system, scout the market by reading consumer magazines or Web sites that test and evaluate these products. One of the best is the Association of Home Appliance Manufacturers (800-267-3138 or *www.cadr.org*). It can help you choose the right air cleaner, tell you where to find replacement filters, and give you the current pollen count in your area.

ALA for diabetes

Super antioxidant stymies pain

ALA or alpha-lipoic acid, found only in tiny amounts in food, makes a big impact on diabetes. It's best known for improving symptoms of diabetic polyneuropathy, a common complication of diabetes that includes painful nerve damage in your feet, legs, and hands. And studies show it can also boost insulin sensitivity.

How it works

Unlike most antioxidants, alpha-lipoic acid works in both fat and water. That, in itself, would be enough to earn a spot on the antioxidant all-star team. But this antioxidant doesn't hog all the glory. Like the best athletes, alpha-lipoic acid also makes its teammates better.

That's because it recycles other antioxidants to make them more effective. When using antioxidants such as vitamins C and E, it's important to also take this little-known coenzyme. It keeps them working at maximum speed, improving sugar metabolism up to 50 percent. The result — a winning team in the fight against diabetes.

Along with its fellow antioxidants, alpha-lipoic acid battles oxidative stress, a major factor in diabetic complications.

Worm your way out of amputation

Medical science has come a long way since the days of maggots and leeches. Or has it?

Even with amazing improvements in technology, diabetic ulcers and other complications still often lead to amputations. But you may be able to avoid losing a limb if you can stomach a creepy alternative.

Doctors in the Netherlands have had success treating diabetic wounds with sterile maggots. Because they only eat dead flesh, maggots are perfect for cleaning out wounds and stopping the spread of infection.

If the sight or sensation of maggots crawling and nibbling on your wound makes you queasy, you can opt for biobags. These porous sacks, filled with maggots, rest on your wound and allow the critters to do their job without actually touching you.

Before agreeing to amputation, ask your doctor about maggot therapy. It may be worth going out on a limb to save yours.

Alpha-lipoic acid also improves microcirculation, or blood flow in the very small blood vessels.

Shows potential

Several studies, mostly from Germany, support the use of alpha-lipoic acid for diabetes. In fact, Germans have been using alpha-lipoic acid to treat polyneuropathy for more than 30 years.

- Studies indicate that taking 600 milligrams (mg) of alpha-lipoic acid, also known as thioctic acid, intravenously for three weeks improves symptoms of neuropathy.

- A small German study showed that taking 1,800 mg of alpha-lipoic acid per day orally for three weeks also helped with symptoms of neuropathy.

- Another German study found that oral alpha-lipoic acid improved insulin sensitivity compared to placebo.

- A Croatian study determined that high doses of alpha-lipoic acid may improve nerve function in people with diabetic polyneuropathy.

Common dosage is 600 mg per day when taken intravenously and 800 mg to 1,800 mg per day when taken orally. Safety does not seem to be an issue.

Right now, alpha-lipoic acid looks like a star-in-waiting, sort of like an elite minor league prospect. But it needs more conclusive long-term studies before it can be recommended without reservations.

Stay tuned

Alpha-lipoic acid has one drawback — it doesn't stay in your bloodstream very long. That's why intravenous alpha-lipoic acid seems more effective than the oral variety. But taking supplements intravenously is not practical, or desirable, for the average person.

Curb diabetic complications

People with diabetes are likely to develop complications. Here's a list of what to watch for early on, and what you can do to prevent problems. By keeping your blood sugar under tight control, you can help prevent all of these conditions.

Watch for	Symptoms	Prevention
diabetic retinopathy	(often without symptoms); floating spots, blurred, or impaired vision	yearly checkup with dilation, daily aspirin
kidney disease	(often without symptoms); high blood pressure	yearly urinary microalbumin test; lower blood pressure with diet and exercise; consider medication
depression	feelings of hopelessness; lack of energy or interest	see your doctor for treatment options
gum disease	red, swollen gums that often bleed when brushed	brush and floss daily; visit dentist twice a year; tell your dentist you have diabetes
osteoporosis	backache; stooped posture; fractures	regular exercise; diet high in potassium, magnesium, vitamins C and D; calcium
carpal tunnel syndrome	numbness, weakness, tingling, or pain in hand or wrist	report pain to your doctor

This problem might be remedied in the future. Taking enteric-coated capsules, which dissolve in your intestines instead of your stomach, or those with a time-released formula might help make alpha-lipoic acid more effective. Keep your eyes open for these products.

Talk with your doctor before taking supplemental alpha-lipoic acid, which may interact with other drugs or supplements designed to do the same thing.

All in all, alpha-lipoic acid looks promising. But, until it's proven conclusively and a more effective oral capsule hits the market, it's a good idea to stick with your current diabetes control program.

Alcohol for insomnia

Sleep better without a nightcap

Think twice about having your favorite alcoholic beverage before heading off to dreamland tonight. Alcohol can make it more difficult for you to fall asleep — and stay asleep.

Unfortunately, you have more to worry about than fatigue if you're not sleeping well. Insomnia can increase your risk for depression, breathing problems, and heart disease.

So if you're having trouble sleeping through the night, try cutting down on alcohol in the evening.

How it works

Chemical messengers in your brain control your sleep stages. Some chemicals slow down brain waves, which allows you to fall asleep. Others stimulate brain waves, causing you to dream and wake up. Alcohol disrupts these normal actions and affects the quality of your sleep.

"In the long run, alcohol isn't the best way to get a good night's sleep," says Dr. Timothy Roehrs, director of research at the Sleep Disorders and Research Center of Henry Ford Hospital.

Conquer insomnia and wake up refreshed

Follow these natural tips, and you'll wake up refreshed and energized in the morning.

- Go to bed and get up at the same time every day.
- Keep your bedroom dark, quiet, and cool.
- Avoid caffeine in the evening.
- Don't eat big meals before bedtime.
- Get regular exercise early in the day.
- Don't drink alcohol in the evening.
- Relax quietly before bedtime with a warm bath.
- Put pets in their own bed. They can disrupt your sleep.
- Get out of bed if you're not sleepy. Read or listen to soft, relaxing music until the sandman returns.

Alcohol stifles dreams

Recently, Roehrs conducted a small study to gauge the effects of alcohol on sleep. His research assistants gave the study participants a placebo or a low dose, one to two glasses, of vodka and tonic water 30 to 60 minutes before bedtime. The placebo provided the illusion of an alcoholic drink by including a few drops of vodka on the surface of the tonic water.

The study showed that alcohol reduced rapid eye movement, or dream sleep, during the first half of the sleep period. What's more — higher doses, three or more glasses, of alcohol increased the number of times the participants woke up during the second half of their sleep period.

Your body metabolizes and eliminates the alcohol during the second half of sleep, causing a rebound effect. In an effort to get back to a normal sleep pattern, the body adjusts to a lack of alcohol by overcorrecting, which causes sleep disruptions.

"Alcohol can seduce people into believing it works, because a small dose of alcohol can initially improve your sleep," says Roehrs. But that's a problem because you quickly develop a tolerance to alcohol within three to seven days. "It makes you believe it's beneficial, then it snatches that benefit away," says Roehrs.

To get around that tolerance and rebound effect, people drink more alcohol, which results in more sleep problems. "We've done studies where we allowed insomniacs to choose the amount of alcohol they wanted before sleep," says Roehrs. "When they were given the chance to take extra drinks, after having the same amount of alcohol for six nights, they automatically increased their dose."

Aging adds to the challenge

You get less and less slow wave or deep sleep as you get older. In fact, many healthy individuals over age 60 will have almost no deep sleep, says Roehrs. This explains why people experience more sleep problems as they get older.

Also, physical challenges, depression, and over-the-counter drugs can cause less-restful deep sleep because you wake more often during the night and early morning.

"As you age, you may sleep less than you use to at night," says Roehrs. "But when you add in the sleep or naps you take during the day, your total amount of sleep for 24 hours may get close to the total amount of sleep you previously had in one night." In the end, your body accepts that.

Antacid gum for heartburn
⭐⭐⭐

Cool down the burning sensation

Many people believe a good meal is one of life's greatest pleasures. Unfortunately, your stomach may not feel the same way. If heartburn is a frequent visitor, here's a little tip — when the burning starts up, cool it down with a simple piece of chewing gum.

How it works

Heartburn is a common symptom of gastroesophageal reflux disease, or GERD. It occurs when stomach acid flows back into your esophagus, the tube that carries food to your stomach. Heartburn is usually at its worst soon after eating a meal, and taking antacids can help reduce the acid levels in your stomach, which relieves uncomfortable symptoms. But if you don't want to overload your system with antacids, try this unusual natural remedy — chewing gum.

Many people find that chewing gum after a meal helps relieve the burning sensation of heartburn. Researchers say this is because the chewing action stimulates the flow of saliva. This naturally alkaline substance neutralizes the acid remaining in your esophagus and helps to wash it away.

Antacid gums take this idea even further by adding an antacid agent, such as calcium carbonate, to the gum. Getting relief from antacids sometimes depends on how long you're exposed to it as well as how well it neutralizes the acid. A gum that releases antacid as it is chewed provides a double whammy and may help relieve your heartburn symptoms faster and for a longer period of time.

Antacid adds an effective twist

To determine the effectiveness of an antacid chewing gum, researchers at the Oklahoma Foundation for Digestive Research separated 24 volunteers into four groups. Each group took either a high-dose antacid gum, a low-dose antacid gum, a chewable antacid tablet, or a placebo.

The study found that when compared with the placebo, both gums decreased heartburn and increased the esophageal pH, balancing out acids from the foods the volunteers had eaten. In fact, both gums provided relief for two hours after the meal. They also worked faster than the chewable antacid and provided longer relief from symptoms.

8 ways to fight heartburn

If heartburn is a frequent guest at your table, use these ideas to make your life more comfortable.

- Eat four to six small meals each day rather than three large ones.
- Drink water throughout the day to keep digestive acids out of your esophagus.
- Cut down on coffee, tea, alcohol, and whole milk. They can irritate your stomach.
- Don't wear your nicotine patch to bed if you're trying to quit smoking. It can cause heartburn.
- Raise the head of your bed 4 to 6 inches to keep your digestive juices flowing downward while you sleep.
- Don't sleep on your back. Sleeping on your left side might reduce your chances of getting heartburn.
- Drink plenty of water with your medications, and don't lie down after swallowing a pill.
- Don't strain or lift heavy items. Your abdominal muscles can squeeze your stomach contents back into your esophagus.

Antacid gum choices

Until recently, Wrigley, the world's largest gum maker, made an antacid gum called *Surpass*. Unfortunately, it did not sell as well as Wrigley expected, and the company took it off the market. You can still find some supplies of *Surpass* at online pharmacy stores, and for sale on e-Bay.

Chooz is another brand of antacid gum that should be in your local pharmacy. If not, ask if they can order it for you through their distributor. You can also go online at *www.americarx.com* or *www.medshopexpress.com* and search for it by name. The average price is $2 to $3 for 16 pieces of gum.

If you can't find antacid gum, use regular gum instead, and chew for about 30 minutes. But be wary of peppermint- or spearmint-flavored gums because they can contribute to heartburn. Peppermint, in particular, may relax the lower ring muscle of your esophagus, allowing stomach acids back in.

If you chew a lot of gum, it's best to use a sugar-free brand to prevent cavities.

Antacids for ulcers

Banish stomach pain for good

You sport a one in 10 chance of developing a peptic ulcer, although having a stressed-out type-A personality won't necessarily improve your chances. Scientists have found ulcers are not caused by stress, but rather by a bacterial infection and possibly long-term use of nonsteroidal anti-inflammatory drugs like aspirin and ibuprofen.

How it works

An ulcer is an open sore in the lining of your stomach or duodenum, the first section of your small intestine. Your stomach secretes powerful acids to digest your food, and these acids irritate the sore when they touch it. Unfortunately, ulcer sufferers seem to produce extra stomach acid, which causes even more discomfort.

That's where antacids may help. They are not quite as effective for ulcers as they are for heartburn, but they can provide some relief since they neutralize acid and raise the pH level of your stomach.

Ulcer healing appears to be related to how much time your stomach pH level stays above 3. Gastric juices are generally in the range of 1.6 to 1.8. When antacids neutralize stomach acid, they help raise your pH to a more acceptable level. Animal studies show that antacids also may have cell-protecting effects.

In the long run, though, cures such as antibiotics to treat *Helicobacter pylori* infection, along with acid-suppressing drugs, are more likely to meet with success.

Try something more effective

New classes of drugs called histamine (H2) receptor antagonists and proton pump inhibitors (PPIs) have pushed antacids out of the running as an ulcer treatment. H2 antagonists, which include the brands Pepcid, Tagamet, and Zantac, work by blocking histamine receptors that give the signal to secrete acid. PPIs like Nexium, Prilosec, and Prevacid block acid production by halting the mechanism that pumps the acid into your stomach.

Research previously showed that PPIs might work better than H2 blockers and antacids for severe gastroesophageal reflux disease (GERD). Now researchers have found they also help heal gastric and duodenal ulcers, particularly when used with antibiotics to combat *H. pylori*.

Monitor your health

One drawback to taking PPIs and H2 blockers may be the small risk of developing pneumonia. In a study of more than 300,000 people, 5,551 cases of pneumonia were diagnosed — 185 of them in people taking acid-suppressing drugs.

Your stomach acid normally kills harmful bacteria. When these drugs suppress the acid, they make it easier for bacteria to multiply. These germs could then get into your lungs and cause pneumonia.

Although noteworthy, this one study does not prove these medications cause pneumonia, and the apparent risk is small. But if you notice breathing problems while taking one of these medications, talk to your doctor about it.

Experts don't know why some people are more susceptible to *H. pylori* infection than others. But one study has shown you may improve your chances of avoiding an ulcer by getting more

Ulcers — the new kissing disease?

Go ahead and kiss your spouse. Even if you have an ulcer.

That may not be something you've worried about, but scientists have. They were concerned the bacteria that cause an ulcer — *Helicobacter pylori* — may spread through kissing after being detected in the saliva of infected people.

However, researchers found no evidence of the bacteria passed on to the spouses of 183 people with suspected ulcers. They identified the bacterium in 16 spouses out of the 89 who definitely had *H. pylori.* But they were different strains that could not have been passed on by the spouse.

Although *H. pylori* commonly resides in the human body, often without causing ulcers, experts don't know how it spreads. They suspect it may be passed through contaminated water and food.

vitamin C into your diet. The study of more than 6,000 adults reported that low blood levels of vitamin C may make a person more likely to become infected by *H. pylori.*

Participants with high blood levels of vitamin C had 11 percent less chance of being infected with the ulcer-causing bacteria.

So drink your orange juice every morning, and include more vitamin C-rich foods like citrus fruits, peppers, and dark leafy greens in your daily menu. They may help you banish stomach pain for good.

Antibacterial soaps for colds

Hand washing keeps you healthy

Cold and flu viruses are often spread by touching, like shaking hands or handling doorknobs. Not surprisingly, experts say washing your hands is one of the most effective ways to fend off those risky viruses.

Judging from TV ads, antibacterial soaps are the best products to use to stop the spread of germs. The advertising must be working. Antibacterial soaps make up three-fourths of all liquid soap sales and nearly a third of all bar soap sales. But do they really deliver on their promise to kill germs?

Not according to the latest studies. Researchers say the kind of soap you use doesn't matter. It's how you wash that makes the difference.

Is it a cold or the flu?		
Symptom	**Cold**	**Flu**
Fever	Rare	Common — begins suddenly, can rise to 102 degrees F to104 degrees F, lasts three to four days
Headache	Rare	Usual
General aches	Slight	Usual — can be quite severe
Fatigue and weakness	Mild	Extreme — can last two to three weeks
Runny, stuffy nose	Common	Sometimes
Sneezing	Usual	Sometimes
Sore throat	Common	Sometimes
Chest discomfort, cough	Mild to moderate, hacking cough	Common — can be severe
Complications	Sinus congestion or earache	Bronchitis, pneumonia, can be life-threatening

How it works

Regular soap works by attacking grime, like dirt, oil, and germs. Its fatty acids bind with the grime, while water droplets capture it. At that point, it's easy to scrub off and wash down the drain.

Antibacterial soaps work the same way except they have an added ingredient, usually triclosan, to kill bacteria. But few people know this antibacterial agent has to remain on your hands for two minutes to do its job.

The next time you wash your hands, see how long you keep them lathered. You'll find you're finished long before two minutes are up. That means you've washed the antibacterial agent down the drain before it could do its job.

Plain old soap works great

A study conducted by researchers at Columbia University in New York deserves special notice. In this study, 238 families made up of 1,178 individuals used unmarked hand washing and cleaning products for a 48-week period.

Half of the participants used antibacterial products, while the other half used regular. The aim of the study was to see if anti-bacterial soap is more effective than regular soap at preventing infectious disease. In the end, the group using antibacterial soap fared no better than those who used regular soap.

One place where lack of proper sanitation can wreak havoc is a cruise ship. Studying the health of people who travel on cruise ships has confirmed the value of washing your hands.

Dr. Robert Wheeler, chairman of the American College of Emergency Physicians' cruise-ship and maritime-medicine sector, says that killing germs involves your hand washing technique, not whether the soap you're using is antibacterial or not. To kill germs on your hands, he says, use soap and warm water, then rub and rinse for 15 seconds. That'll do it.

Be choosy at the store

Viruses, not bacteria, cause colds and flu. Antibacterial products kill bacteria, not viruses.

And experts say these soaps can actually do more harm than good. They're probably killing just as many good bacteria as bad, and creating antibiotic-resistant super bugs in the process.

What's more, many scientists are concerned about the long-term environmental effects of washing antibacterial soaps down the drain.

As if that's not enough, waterless antibacterial cleaners and wipes are mainly alcohol — flammable and potentially dangerous.

Antibiotics for Crohn's disease

Zap hidden cause of IBD

Like pirates seeking buried treasure, scientists seek a cure for Crohn's disease. Now some researchers believe they've found the map — or, rather MAP, as in *Mycobacterium avium paratuberculosis,* a type of bacteria that may cause this inflammatory bowel disease (IBD).

The theory is similar to the recent breakthrough in treating ulcers. Long blamed on stress and spicy foods, ulcers actually have a much more sinister cause — *H. pylori.* Get rid of the bacteria, and you get rid of the ulcer.

Just as antibiotics clear up ulcers, they may also help people with Crohn's disease.

How it works

Crohn's disease is a chronic illness that affects your digestive tract, usually your lower small intestine or colon. Although the cause of the disease is unknown, one theory is that it is brought on by environmental factors, such as diet and smoking, in people with a family history of the disease.

Some researchers also think certain types of bacteria that grow in low temperatures may contribute to Crohn's. These "psychrotrophic" bacteria often develop in meats and cheeses found in your refrigerator. The bacterium *M. paratuberculosis* has been found to infect cows and may pass to you through their milk.

These, or other viruses or bacteria, may trigger an autoimmune reaction against your gastrointestinal tract.

One way antibiotics help relieve Crohn's disease is to wipe out these bacteria. Studies have also found they can close abnormal channels called fistulas that develop between parts of your bowel or between your bowel and other organs. This provides some relief while giving immune-suppressing drugs time to work.

Combo squelches flareups

Much of the evidence in support of antibiotics comes from small, open-label trials. While they can provide clues for future research, they lack the weight of large, randomized, double-blind, placebo-controlled trials.

- The combination of rifabutin and clarithromycin or azithromycin, a new generation of antibiotics, worked well in a preliminary British trial. Nearly 94 percent of those in the study went into remission. Two-thirds remained in remission for two years.

- Australian researchers used rifabutin, clarithromycin, and clofazimine to treat 12 people with severe Crohn's disease. Six went into complete remission, while others saw improvement.

- A University of Central Florida study had similar success with rifabutin, clarithromycin, and a probiotic supplement. About 58 percent of the people in the study reached a sustained state of improvement. Others improved, but needed other drugs to stay healthy.

- University of Central Florida researchers also showed that the presence of anti-MAP antibodies p35 and p36 in the blood can successfully diagnose Crohn's disease, which can be tricky to differentiate from ulcerative colitis.

- In an Austrian study, half the people saw improvement in fistula activity after eight weeks of antibiotic therapy with ciprofloxacin and metronidazole. But the immune-suppressing drug azathioprine was needed to maintain improvement.

Keep in mind these studies are preliminary. It's too early to proclaim antibiotics a success — but they look promising.

Work with your doctor

Different researchers used different amounts of the antibiotics in their studies. You'll need to work with your doctor to determine the particular dosage.

All of these antibiotics come with possible side effects you should know about.

- Side effects of rifabutin and clarithromycin treatment included yellowing or reddening of the skin, fatigue, and joint pain.

- With ciprofloxacin, you might experience sensitivity to sunlight.

- Metronidazole may cause nausea, diarrhea, and a sharp metallic taste.

You can't do antibiotic therapy on your own. You'll need a prescription and a doctor's guidance. But you can bring the possible MAP link to your doctor's attention.

Another step you can take is to heat your milk to kill any possible MAP bacteria. To be safe, use a kitchen thermometer and make sure the milk reaches 176 to 185 degrees Fahrenheit. Then let it cool before using it.

It may help to eat several small meals throughout the day instead

> Some experts believe people with Crohn's disease could benefit from increasing their intake of antioxidant vitamins — such as vitamins E and C.

of three large ones. Cutting out spicy or fatty foods may also help you avoid problems.

Don't give up on standard treatments for Crohn's, which include steroids, mesalamine, and immune-suppressing drugs. But keep your eyes open for new developments involving antibiotics.

You just might make Crohn's disease walk the plank.

Anti-cellulite creams for cellulite

No magic cure for 'dimpled' skin

Let's face it — cellulite looks bad. This lumpy fat under the skin of your thighs, hips, and buttocks gives your skin a dimpled look often compared to an orange peel.

Cellulite mostly affects women, who are bombarded with advertisements for creams, gels, and lotions that promise to make it disappear.

But there's no magic cure in these anti-cellulite creams. In fact, they're much better at removing money from your pocketbook than cellulite from your thighs.

How it works

Cellulite likely develops when small blood vessels in the fatty tissue under the skin become damaged, causing circulation to slow and fluid to accumulate.

How — or whether — creams work depends on their ingredients. Some drugs, like caffeine or aminophylline, boast fat-splitting powers. Others may affect microcirculation, or blood flow in small blood vessels. But mostly, creams just soften your skin.

A Finnish study examined the ingredients of 32 cellulite creams. Various herbs and emollients, or skin softeners, made up the bulk of the 263 ingredients. The most common active ingredient was caffeine. All creams included some kind of fragrance, and nearly every product contained between 50 to 90 percent water.

Strong on hype, weak on proof

Few good scientific studies have been done to support the claims of anti-cellulite creams.

- A study by England's Bradford Royal Infirmary showed that topical aminophylline does not work. After applying either a 2-percent aminophylline cream or a placebo twice a day for 12 weeks, participants noticed improvement in only three of 35 treated legs. Also, 24 percent of the women in the study developed a rash.

- Hope exists for topical retinol. A Belgian study found that retinol helps smooth skin, echoing the results of an earlier study by the University of Pennsylvania School of Medicine. However, both studies were small, and more trials are needed.

Researchers have a tough time because there's no standard method for judging a treatment's success. In addition, other factors, such as weight loss, diet, and exercise, play such a big role. But what anti-cellulite creams lack in proof, they more than make up for in hype.

Save your money

To get the most out of anti-cellulite cream, you'll have to apply it over wide areas of skin every morning and evening for at least two months. This can be very expensive, since products can cost as much as $50 for just a few ounces. That's a lot of money to waste for meager results.

While anti-cellulite creams seem safe for most people, they do include some ingredients that may cause allergic reactions. Fragrances, preservatives, or plant extracts are the most common culprits.

If you want to try anti-cellulite cream, it shouldn't be too hard to find. In fact, it will probably find you. Just keep your eyes open for ads in women's magazines or spam in your e-mail inbox. You can also find it in hair salons, drugstores, or on the Internet.

Several other cellulite treatments are available, including different types of massage, electromagnetic fields, herbal supplements, or even liposuction. None of these are recommended, either. Your best bet is to lose weight and exercise.

Remember, cellulite will not magically disappear. But if you fall for anti-cellulite gimmicks, your money will.

Tone up for firmer skin

The only way to get rid of cellulite is to get rid of those fat cells lurking under your skin. And to do that you must lose some weight and tone up your muscles.

- Eat a healthy, balanced diet.
- Work out with light weights or resistance bands.
- Target problem areas with specific exercises. For instance, leg lifts or raises are particularly good for your buttocks and thighs.

Aromatherapy for stress

Calm anxiety with essential oils

Imagine the delightful scent of lavender or the inviting aroma of cedar. Powerful essential oils in the lavender plant and cedar tree are the source of those fragrances, and they can help relieve anxiety and stress.

How it works

Aromatherapy uses the scents from plants, herbs, and flowers to heal the mind and body. This age-old remedy enhances feelings of well-being.

Your sense of smell is linked to your limbic system, the part of the brain involved in memory and emotion. That means if you smell something pleasant and familiar, it may evoke a pleasant, relaxing sensation because it has stimulated the alpha brainwaves associated with relaxation.

In a study, researchers found that inhaling the aroma of essential oils did not lessen pain or change peoples' physical responses to pain. However, it did soften the participants' negative memory of a painful event. Researchers have found that lavender oils, in particular, may help lessen stress and anxiety during painful experiences.

Sniff out more evidence

Aromatherapy research has been sparse, but these studies suggest it may be more than just good scents.

- Researchers found that people who sniffed a floral fragrance during dental appointments stayed more relaxed.
- Two small studies suggest lavender and lemon balm essential oils may help calm agitation in people with dementia.

- A study at the University of Miami School of Medicine found that just three minutes of aromatherapy with lavender scent were relaxing and eased depression.

Meanwhile, the cosmetics industry is researching which fragrances make the best stress-reducing bubble bath and which ones can relax tight muscles between your shoulder blades when you're tense. But aromatherapy still needs large, independently funded trials to help prove whether it works.

Make every drop count

Before you buy an essential oil, check the Latin botanical name on the container. Several different species of a plant may go by the same common name, but an herb's strength and healing power may vary from one species to another. These oils are known to relieve anxiety and stress.

Find serenity with simple changes

Fine-tune the priorities in your life and you could feel stress taking a back seat to tranquility. Try to make at least some of these activities part of your everyday routine.

- Stretch.
- Exercise.
- Get enough quality sleep.
- Practice conscious breathing — take slow, deep breaths.
- Laugh.
- Get a pet.
- Let go of fear, anger, guilt, and sadness.
- Eat well to stay healthy.
- Pray.
- Spend time with loved ones.
- Get a massage.
- Listen to soothing music.

- bergamot (*Citrus bergamia*)
- cedarwood (*Cedrus atlantica*)
- frankincense (*Boswellia carteri*)
- geranium (*Pelargonium graveolens*)
- hyssop (*Hyssopus officinalis*)
- lavender (*Lavendula officinalis* or *Lavendula angustifolia*)
- sandalwood (*Santalum album*)
- ylang ylang (*Canaga odorata*)

Relax and enjoy these amazing stress-busters.

- Run a steamy bath and add five to 10 drops of essential oil and one ounce of carrier oil. Soak for at least 15 minutes.
- For a stress headache, soak a hand towel in a mixture of a half-cup of water and five to 10 drops of essential oil. Hold the compress to your forehead until the towel is cold.
- For the perfect massage, add 10 to 20 drops of essential oil to every one ounce of carrier oil. But if you use citrus oils, stay out of the sun. These oils can make your skin extra-sensitive to sunlight.
- Dab a handkerchief with three to four drops of your favorite essential oil. Sniff it at arm's length for instant stress relief.
- Enjoy a 10-minute footbath with hot water and a few drops of essential oil.

Remember to keep essential oils out of your mouth and eyes and never place undiluted essential oils directly on your skin. Always dilute them in water or "carrier oils," like almond, apricot, jojoba, and grapeseed.

Store essential oils in dark, tightly sealed containers. Keep them in a cool, dry place out of reach of children and pets.

Artichoke leaf extract for high cholesterol

Tell cholesterol to take a hike

You've changed your diet to lower cholesterol, but you've heard artichokes may coax your cholesterol readings even closer to normal. Scientists have been studying the extract of artichoke leaves to determine if this is true. Here's what they've learned.

How it works

Artichoke leaf extract may attack cholesterol in two ways. Not only could it help sweep out the cholesterol you're stuck with now, but it may also limit the new cholesterol your body makes.

Operation Sweep-Out-Cholesterol begins in your liver. Bile from your liver helps break down cholesterol from the fat you eat. These fatty particles are transported to the intestines where enzymes can digest them. So more bile may mean less cholesterol in your bloodstream. But a liver that doesn't produce enough bile lets too much cholesterol slip by. That's where artichoke leaf extract may help. The extract seems to stimulate the liver into producing more bile.

An artichoke leaf compound called cynarin may be the driving force behind bile's cholesterol sweep-out. In fact, cynarin extract has been used in cholesterol-lowering drugs.

But that's not all. Artichoke leaves may also help keep new cholesterol from forming in your liver. One animal study suggests that luteolin — an ingredient in artichoke leaves — might cut cholesterol production.

Follow this promising story

In one high cholesterol study, some participants received artichoke juice instead of cholesterol-lowering drugs. Their bad LDL cholesterol, total cholesterol, and triglyceride levels fell an average of 8 percent, while their good HDL cholesterol levels rose. The people taking traditional medicines lowered their cholesterol levels only a few percentage points more.

A German study showed that 1,800 milligrams of dry artichoke extract daily caused LDL cholesterol to fall by more than 22 percent. Total cholesterol dropped by 18 percent. But this study only tested 143 people for six weeks. A review of the research on artichoke leaf extract concluded that larger and longer-lasting studies are needed before scientists can tell us just how safe and effective this extract really is.

Learn the good and the bad

The good news is studies on artichoke leaf extract don't seem to find any dangerous or lasting side effects. The extract might act as a mild diuretic, and one study reported mild effects like

End indigestion with artichoke leaf extract

Artichoke leaf extract isn't just a potential cholesterol fighter. It may help end indigestion, too. If you feel sick to your stomach, overly full, and have abdominal pain — even though you ate a normal-sized meal — you may suffer from dyspepsia. That's a fancy name for poor digestion.

Several studies showed dramatic improvements in people with dyspepsia after they were treated with artichoke extracts. These folks might have experienced the same bile shortage that's been blamed for boosting cholesterol. After all, if the liver doesn't produce enough bile, food doesn't get broken down properly — and then the stomach pains and indigestion set in. But ingredients in artichokes can help the liver form bile so digestion runs smoothly again.

hunger, flatulence, or weakness. But several studies reported no side effects at all.

In spite of this, some people shouldn't touch artichoke leaf extract with a 10-foot pole. Avoid it completely if you have a bile duct obstruction, artichoke allergies, or allergies to any member of the daisy family. Steer clear of products labeled "*Cynara* extract" or "*Cynara scolymus* extract" too. If you have gallstones or gall bladder disease, get your doctor's approval before you try this extract.

If you do decide to take it, follow the directions on the label. Dosages of 1.5 grams (1,500 milligrams) per day of the dry extract successfully lowered cholesterol in one study. Tinctures,

7 easy ways to bring down high cholesterol

By controlling your cholesterol, you decrease your risk of developing all kinds of heart-related problems, including atherosclerosis and high blood pressure. Here's what every person can do to keep those cholesterol numbers where they should be.

- Eat more garlic.
- Increase the amount of fiber in your diet. Whole grains and fresh fruits and vegetables slash cholesterol and fill you up.
- Get less saturated fat — like from red meat, butter, and palm oil.
- Maintain a healthy weight.
- Eat several small meals throughout the day instead of three large ones. This keeps hormones, like insulin, from rising and signaling your body to make cholesterol. Just don't increase your total calories.
- Exercise regularly.
- Load up on fruits and vegetables containing the antioxidant vitamins E and C — dark leafy greens and brightly colored produce.

fluid extracts, and artichoke juice may also be available at the health food store, but the correct dosage is different for each one.

Researchers have not pinpointed any drug interactions with artichoke leaf extract, but keep an eye on new research to be sure. If you take prescription or over-the-counter medications — especially cholesterol-lowering drugs — play it safe. Talk with your doctor before trying this remedy.

Aspirin for Alzheimer's

Pain relievers might prevent AD

A "vaccine" that prevents deadly Alzheimer's disease? These popular little pills could be the answer. Best of all, you may already take them for everyday aches. Aspirin, ibuprofen, and other nonsteroidal anti-inflammatory drugs (NSAIDs) not only ease inflammation — they may also protect you from Alzheimer's disease (AD).

In fact, people with rheumatoid arthritis are up to 12 times less likely to develop Alzheimer's. Could the NSAIDs they take for their arthritis hold the key?

How it works

Brain inflammation is a hallmark of Alzheimer's disease. Researchers think beta-amyloid, a toxic substance, gradually builds up in the brains of people who have AD and

> Want even more protection from Alzheimer's? Exercise and stop smoking.

triggers inflammation. This, in turn, damages more brain cells. NSAIDs don't stop this toxic accumulation, but they do break the inflammatory chain reaction.

Here's how it happens. The foods you eat provide your body with arachidonic acid. Once in your system, this essential fatty acid attaches to the enzyme cyclooxygenase-2 (COX-2). This enzyme uses arachidonic acid to make a hormone called prostaglandin, the main culprit in inflammation.

NSAIDs keep COX-2 from producing prostaglandin. They temporarily plug up the hole on the enzyme where arachidonic acid attaches, like sticking a cork into a bottle. Eventually the effect wears off, and you have to take another dose.

Aspirin seems to work differently, but experts aren't sure exactly how. It may permanently neutralize the COX-2 enzyme, reducing pain and swelling until your body makes new enzymes.

NSAIDs not only ease pain and swelling, they also thin your blood. Some experts believe these drugs might protect against

Eat right to avoid AD

Is your diet giving you Alzheimer's? Don't lose your mind to old age. Learn the keys to keeping your brain in tip-top shape with foods that keep your memory healthy. Start these strategies now to prevent Alzheimer's later.

- Go low-fat. A diet high in saturated fat and trans fatty acids could double your risk for AD. Cut back on margarine, switch to lean meat, and load up on the AD-fighting fats in fish, olive oil, and avocados, instead.
- Eat your Bs. B12, niacin, and folate, that is. These brainy vitamins may protect you from Alzheimer's. Look for B12 in lean meat and low-fat dairy, and niacin in legumes, nuts, and tea. Leafy greens and broccoli are full of folate.
- Add apples. Apples and apple juice may act as an antioxidant, thereby protecting brain cells from damaging oxidation that contributes to AD. Choose juices low in added sugar.

AD not so much by reducing inflammation as by improving blood flow in your brain.

NSAIDs show promise

Past research has yielded mixed results. Some studies have linked NSAID use to lower AD risk, while others have not.

One group of scientists recently set out to settle the debate. They pooled the results of nine studies involving more than 16,000 people over the last 35 years. They examined the protective effects of NSAIDs as a group, then analyzed aspirin separately.

Overall, NSAIDs showed promise in preventing AD. What's more — the longer you take them, the more you may lower your risk.

- People who took them for less than a month decreased their danger of developing Alzheimer's by 5 percent.

- Those who took them for less than two years saw a 17-percent decline in their risk.

- People who took NSAIDs for more than two years snagged the biggest benefit — an amazing 73-percent drop in their chances of developing AD.

- Aspirin alone reduced the risk of Alzheimer's disease by 13 percent.

Aspirin did not seem to fend off AD as well as other NSAIDs. These researchers say not enough studies have been done on aspirin's role in Alzheimer's. Keep in mind it works differently, and this may affect how well it protects against AD.

> Take NSAIDs with food to ease their unpleasant side effects, unless your doctor says otherwise.

NSAIDs may help prevent Alzheimer's, but they will not cure it. A major study funded by the National Institutes of Health found they do not slow the progress of the disease once it takes hold. Scientists tested a placebo against low doses of two NSAIDs, naproxen and rofecoxib, in people with mild Alzheimer's disease. These two drugs worked no better than the sugar pill at putting the brakes on advancing AD.

Take with a dose of caution

Experts still don't know how much you need of any NSAID to build your defense against Alzheimer's. Some studies suggest the dosages people take to ease arthritis may do the trick. Just remember — questions still stand about if and how these pills prevent AD, and more research is underway.

The grape debate

In the past few years, several studies have suggested drinking wine in moderate amounts may lower some people's risk of Alzheimer's disease.

The grapes may hold the key. Some scientists think eating grapes or drinking grape juice might have the same protective effect as wine, without the dangers of alcohol.

Dr. Michael Seidman, director of the Otologic/Neurotologic Surgery Division and medical director for the Center for Integrative Medicine at Henry Ford Health System likes the idea but isn't sure grapes alone would do the trick. "I don't have the complete answer at this time, but I do believe alcohol has an effect."

However, he says straight alcohol, like grain alcohol, probably won't work. Neither, he believes, would resveratrol, an antioxidant in grape skins. "I think it's a combination of the tannins, the antioxidants, the resveratrol, and the alcohol." Rather than one factor alone, all of these things might play a part.

In the meantime, talk with your doctor before you begin using aspirin, ibuprofen, or other NSAID regularly. These drugs thin your blood and can cause internal bleeding, ulcers, and other serious side effects, especially when used long-term. You should only take them under your doctor's supervision.

Aspirin for breast cancer

Headache remedy battles cancer

Aspirin might be the next line of defense against cancer. Early studies suggest taking these pills could slash your risk of breast cancer, particularly for women at high risk of certain types of breast cancer.

How it works

In the last few years, scientists have spent more time studying chemopreventive therapies, drugs like tamoxifen that prevent breast cancer or its recurrence. Now experts suspect one cheap, common pill may hold similar preventive powers.

Studies have found that aspirin, along with ibuprofen and other nonsteroidal anti-inflammatory drugs (NSAIDs), may limit the development and growth of tumors in the breast.

Their role in preventing breast cancer is thought to stem from their ability to block the enzyme cyclo-oxygenase (COX) 2. This enzyme produces substances called prostaglandins that promote inflammation and could be involved in the process of tumor development.

Prostaglandins also stimulate an enzyme critical to the pro-duction of the hormones estrogen and progesterone. Women at risk of hormone-receptor positive breast cancer, the most common kind among older women, may benefit the most from NSAID therapy.

In this type, the cancerous tumors feed on estrogen or progesterone. Researchers theorize that by blocking COX-2, aspirin may help lower these hormone levels in your blood and prevent tumors from developing.

Future protection for NSAID-users

Aspirin has seemed to prevent breast cancer in animal studies and some human studies, but other human studies show no protective effect. Scientists may finally be unraveling this mystery with the completion of two recent epidemiological studies, both of which point to the cancer-quelling power of NSAIDs.

The Women's Health Initiative Observational Study surveyed over 80,000 postmenopausal women between the ages of 50 and 79 with no history of cancer, asking them how often they

---

Raise your defenses against breast cancer

Don't be afraid of breast cancer. Learn all you can about how to protect yourself from it and how to fight it. Start by talking to your doctor and practicing these important tips now.

- Get a mammogram.
- Conduct a breast self-exam every month.
- Watch your weight.
- Cook with monounsaturated fats — like olive and canola oil — instead of polyunsaturated fats — like corn, safflower, and sunflower oil.
- Limit your alcohol intake.
- Exercise regularly.
- Get more antioxidant vitamins through a variety of fresh fruits and vegetables.
- Add flaxseed to your diet.

---

used aspirin, ibuprofen, other NSAIDs, and acetaminophen. Researchers then followed up with the women twice a year to find out who developed breast cancer.

Women who took NSAIDs regularly, two or more pills per week, had the least chance of getting breast cancer, and the longer they took it, the more benefit they reaped.

- Women taking NSAIDs regularly for five to nine years reduced their risk by 21 percent.

- Those who took it regularly for 10 or more years dropped it even more, by 28 percent.

- Ibuprofen seemed to offer more protection than aspirin.

- Acetaminophen, on the other hand, had no effect, nor did low doses of aspirin, such as baby aspirin.

The Long Island Breast Cancer study, a new observational study, found similar benefits. Women who took aspirin at least seven times a week had the lowest risk of hormone-receptor positive breast cancer, 28 percent lower than other women.

Ibuprofen, however, had a weaker effect in this study, dropping the risk of this kind of cancer by 22 percent in women who took it less than three times a week.

NSAIDs, in general, had little effect on hormone-receptor negative cancer. Experts believe these findings confirm their theory as to why NSAIDs may protect some women from breast cancer.

Standby for further results

Similar studies have linked aspirin and other NSAIDs to a decreased risk of several types of cancer, including colorectal cancer. But experts argue it's too early to tell women to take NSAIDs regularly.

Good clinical trials in the future will help researchers better understand if and how these drugs fight breast cancer, and what dosages women should take to maximize their benefit.

In the meantime, if you already take an NSAID for heart health or arthritis, you may also be shoring yourself up against certain kinds of cancer. Use these drugs with caution. They can lead to ulcers and gastrointestinal bleeding, as well as thin your blood.

Enteric-coated NSAIDs tend to be easier on your stomach, and taking them with food can also ease the stomach upset they sometimes cause.

Aspirin for stroke prevention

★★★

Daily pill drop kicks risk

Stroke strikes someone every minute.

That means a blood vessel becomes blocked (ischemic) or bursts (hemorrhagic), cutting off blood flow to part of your brain. Without the oxygen in the blood, your brain cells die — and never come back. Depending on which part of your brain is affected, you could be paralyzed on one side of your body, lose feeling, balance, bladder control, or sight, or have trouble swallowing, talking, or remembering things. Of course, stroke can also kill you.

You have to be extra cautious as you get older. Two-thirds of all stroke victims are over 65 years old. In fact, your risk of stroke doubles every decade after you turn 55.

Just thinking about it is enough to give you a headache. Luckily, the same simple remedy — aspirin — will improve both your head and your chances of avoiding a stroke.

Strike at the 'heart' of strokes

Don't become one of the 15 million stroke victims this year. A few easy lifestyle changes could make all the difference to your heart.

- Stop smoking. It contributes to a build-up of fatty substances that can block the main artery supplying blood to your brain.
- Exercise regularly. This helps keep your blood pressure under control, reducing your risk of stroke.
- Eat at least five servings of fruits and vegetables a day. Cruciferous vegetables, like broccoli, cabbage, and cauliflower; green leafy vegetables; and citrus fruits and juices seem to have the greatest protective effect.
- Get more B vitamins through your diet or supplements. They help control a substance called homocysteine that can damage and narrow your arteries.
- Eat cold-water, fatty fish — like salmon, sardines, herring, and mackerel — a few times a week.
- Moderate your alcohol intake — especially beer.

How it works

Aspirin may be the safest, cheapest, most effective way to fight stroke and heart attack. Salicylic acid, the active part of aspirin, is an antiplatelet agent. That means it decreases the stickiness of blood platelets, which helps prevent them from clumping together to form clots. Since blood clots are a primary cause of stroke, aspirin therapy is often prescribed for people at high risk, particularly those who have suffered a previous minor stroke.

Beats expensive drugs

Aspirin's effectiveness has been proven in several clinical trials. A review of more than 100 studies determined that aspirin slashes the risk of future strokes by 25 to 30 percent in people who have had a minor stroke or a transient ischemic attack (TIA).

Strokes per year in the United States	
Men	327,000
Women	373,000
Total	700,000

In fact, aspirin worked better than ticlopidine, a much more expensive antiplatelet drug, in a study of black men and women who had recently suffered a stroke.

Right now, experts do not advise healthy people over age 50 who have not had a stroke or TIA to take aspirin as a preventive measure.

Dodge the dangers

Just one tablet of aspirin a day, ranging from 81 mg to 325 mg, should give you the protection you need. But aspirin therapy comes with some drawbacks. Common side effects include stomach pain, heartburn, indigestion, nausea, and vomiting. You also run the risk of more serious side effects, such as peptic ulcers, gastrointestinal bleeding, and hemorrhagic stroke, the kind caused by bleeding in the brain.

If you have high blood pressure, get it under control before beginning aspirin therapy. Proceed with caution — or reconsider aspirin therapy — if you take other NSAIDs, particularly ibuprofen, or anticoagulant drugs. The combination can limit the protective effects of aspirin or increase the risk of serious side effects.

Aspirin therapy may not work for everyone. Some people are resistant to aspirin. A recent study found that these people were three times as likely to have a stroke or heart attack or die as those who respond to aspirin.

You can buy aspirin pretty much anywhere — pharmacies, supermarkets, convenience stores. Just make sure to consult your doctor before beginning aspirin therapy.

If aspirin doesn't work for you, other antiplatelet drugs such as ticlopidine or clopidogrel, or anticoagulant medication, might be better options.

Exercising regularly, losing weight, quitting smoking, and eating a healthy diet low in fat and salt and high in fruits, vegetables, and fiber will also help you avoid a stroke.

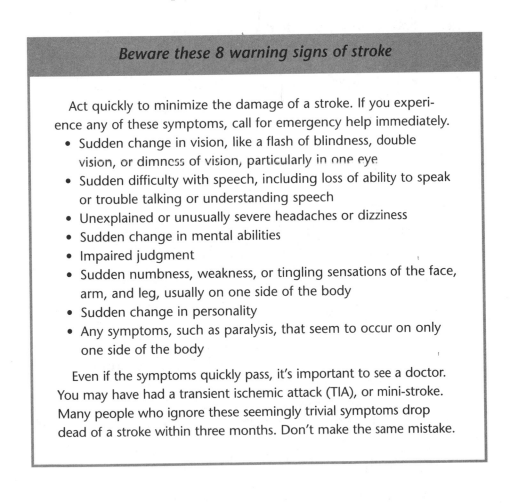

Beware these 8 warning signs of stroke

Act quickly to minimize the damage of a stroke. If you experience any of these symptoms, call for emergency help immediately.

- Sudden change in vision, like a flash of blindness, double vision, or dimness of vision, particularly in one eye
- Sudden difficulty with speech, including loss of ability to speak or trouble talking or understanding speech
- Unexplained or unusually severe headaches or dizziness
- Sudden change in mental abilities
- Impaired judgment
- Sudden numbness, weakness, or tingling sensations of the face, arm, and leg, usually on one side of the body
- Sudden change in personality
- Any symptoms, such as paralysis, that seem to occur on only one side of the body

Even if the symptoms quickly pass, it's important to see a doctor. You may have had a transient ischemic attack (TIA), or mini-stroke. Many people who ignore these seemingly trivial symptoms drop dead of a stroke within three months. Don't make the same mistake.

B vitamins for depression

★★☆

Nutrients help lift your spirits

Childhood memories of having to eat liver and spinach might be depressing thoughts, but it should be just the opposite. Both foods are full of folate, one of several important B vitamins that can help lift you out of depression.

The exact connection isn't clear, but experts know depression gets worse when people are deficient in folate and seems to improve when levels are high.

Vitamin B12 works closely with folate. Many signs of deficiency, including depression, are the same for both vitamins. Lack of vitamins B1 (thiamin) and B6 are also associated with depression.

How it works

Carbohydrate, protein, and fat give your body fuel for energy. The B vitamins help your body use this fuel. Most of the time, you don't even notice them, but when they're not working, you can suffer a multitude of symptoms, including exhaustion, irritability, forgetfulness, and depression.

Folate and vitamin B12 are the Bs most commonly associated with depression. They work with B6 to help produce neurotransmitters — chemicals that carry messages between your nerves and brain. Thiamin helps nerve signals travel from your brain to all parts of your body.

B vitamins are important in many ways:

- Nerve processes depend heavily on thiamin, which is also essential for energy metabolism in all cells.

- Brain development and function depend on vitamin B6, and it keeps nerve and muscle cells healthy. It also might help relieve stress and some premenstrual syndrome (PMS) symptoms.

- Nerve fibers become damaged without vitamin B12, which helps maintain the sheaths that protect them.

- New cells and DNA are formed with the help of folate. It also helps your body make serotonin, a neurotransmitter that produces feelings of calmness and contentment.

Research targets folate

Recent studies from Norway and Tufts University in Boston have associated low folate levels with depression. Researchers also found that lack of vitamin B12 plays a role because of the way the two B vitamins work together.

A big unanswered question is whether low folate levels actually cause depression or if results of depression — such as loss of appetite — lead to lower folate intake.

Ingvar Bjelland, a medical doctor and Ph.D. at the University of Bergen in Norway, was the lead researcher in one study. He

---

Escape this common menace

A simple vitamin B12 deficiency can cause loss of balance, muscle weakness, incontinence, moodiness, and dementia. This easily treated disorder is hard to detect because routine blood tests probably won't tell your doctor you have it.

More often than not, a vitamin B12 deficiency means you're not absorbing it from the foods you eat, especially if you're over age 60. It's important to see your doctor for a proper diagnosis.

If you have this disorder, you might be able to get enough extra B12 from fortified foods and supplements. However, in some cases, your doctor may recommend vitamin B12 injections.

Pep up your step with B vitamins

Do you feel tired and sluggish, even though you're not sick? Maybe you need more B vitamins. These common nutrients don't actually supply energy directly to your body. Instead, they act as co-enzymes that help unlock energy-producing fuel from the food you eat.

Active forms of the B vitamins thiamin, riboflavin, niacin, pantothenic acid, and biotin all help release energy from carbohydrates, fats, and protein. Vitamin B6 assists in converting amino acids into protein, and vitamin B12 and folate are important in building and repairing new cells — especially red blood cells.

B vitamins might help you feel better and have more energy in a matter of weeks. Foods that supply them include meat, dairy products, whole grains, nuts, and leafy green vegetables. If you think you aren't getting enough, ask your doctor if you should take a B-complex supplement.

---

thinks it's more probable that low folate levels cause depression, but he won't go so far as to say that stepping up folate levels will help relieve it.

"We don't actually know if folate itself really helps fighting depression," he says. "Most studies are looking at folate as a supplement to conventional antidepressants."

Folate helps some drugs used to treat depression work better. Bjelland, a specialist in psychiatry, says maybe it's because of folate's relationship to serotonin. Antidepressants work by increasing serotonin levels in the brain.

A study of 115 people suffering with depression — all outpatients at a hospital in Finland — found that those who had high levels of vitamin B12 in their blood responded better to treatment. Experts think it could be because folate needs vitamin B12 to work more efficiently.

Best bet for B vitamins

Food is your best source of B vitamins because in addition to these nutrients, you'll get other important vitamins and minerals, too. You can't stay healthy if you overload on a single vitamin.

Legumes and whole grains provide vitamin B6, thiamin, and folate; B12 and B6 are found in meats; leafy green vegetables provide folate and B6; liver is a rich source of B12, thiamin, and folate; and a baked potato yields both B6 and thiamin.

B vitamins for breakfast				
Ready-to-eat cereal	**Amount per cup**			
	Thiamin	**Folate**	**Vitamin B6**	**Vitamin B12**
General Mills Whole Grain Total	2.8 mg	1076 mcg	3.8 mg	8.6 mcg
Kellogg's Special K	.5 mg	676 mcg	2 mg	6.1 mcg
Kellogg's Complete Wheat Bran Flakes	2.1 mg	909 mcg	2 mg	8 mcg
Kellogg's Product 19	1.5 mg	676 mcg	2 mg	6 mcg
General Mills Total Raisin Bran	1.5 mg	673 mcg	2 mg	6 mcg
RDA for men over age 50	*1.2 mg*	*400 mcg*	*1.7 mg*	*2.4 mcg*
RDA for women over age 50	*1.1 mg*	*400 mcg*	*1.5 mg*	*2.4 mcg*

In the United States, enriched grain products, such as bread and cereal, are now fortified with extra folate. Older people sometimes need supplements because they don't absorb B vitamins — especially vitamin B12 — from food very well.

Check with a nutritionist or doctor before taking large doses of supplements. It's almost impossible to get too many B vitamins from food, but if you overdo supplements, you could experience serious side effects.

B vitamins for osteoporosis

New way to battle brittle bones

When you're thinking about vitamins, remember "B for bones." It's possible that certain B vitamins can help strengthen your bones and prevent osteoporosis.

Two recent studies suggest that high levels of the amino acid homocysteine is linked with broken bones. The good news is B vitamins help get rid of homocysteine.

How it works

The amino acid homocysteine is made from another amino acid, methionine, to help metabolize protein. When the process is complete, homocysteine should be turned back into methionine, but here's the catch. It needs B vitamins to be converted back to its original form.

If you don't have enough B vitamins to do the job, homocysteine can build up to dangerous levels, causing damage to your arteries — and possibly osteoporosis.

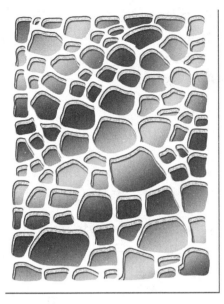

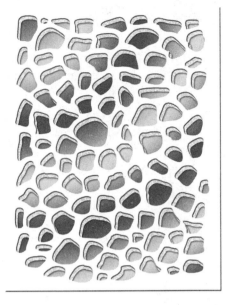

This is what bone looks like when viewed with a microscope. You can see the trabecula – the interlaced rods of bone tissue that form a web or network to help make bones strong. But in this picture, osteoporosis has thinned the trabecula, widening the spaces between them and making the bone more brittle.

When normal bone is viewed under a microscope, you see thick trabecula with smaller spaces between them – a sure sign of stronger bones.

Researchers aren't exactly sure what the connection between homocysteine and osteoporosis is. This is what they've come up with so far.

- Homocysteine interferes with the ability of collagen to hold bones together.

- Since homocysteine is also linked with heart disease and weakened mental ability, people with these conditions may be more frail and fall down more often.

- Increased homocysteine might only be an indicator of poor nutrition. Other studies have shown that older women with a vitamin B12 deficiency are more prone to bone loss and fractures.

Beef up on B12

Whether it's the homocysteine or the lack of nutrients that's the problem, it will help if you make sure you're getting enough B vitamins — and the best one to get in this case is B12.

"Homocysteine is a necessary part of metabolism," says Sally Stabler, medical doctor and professor of medicine at the University of Colorado Health Sciences Center. "Studies have shown that high levels of homocysteine are harmful in themselves, but high homocysteine can also point to vitamin B12 deficiency."

Stabler, a leading researcher of homocysteine and B vitamins, says both vitamin B12 and folate are needed to change homocysteine into methionine.

"In the United States and Canada, people are eating a lot of folate in fortified grain products," she says. "Therefore, high homocysteine is usually due to B12 deficiency. B6 is not usually a problem."

Bone up on osteoporosis prevention

A recent Surgeon General's report says weak and broken bones should no longer be considered a normal part of old age. You can have strong bones and avoid osteoporosis all your life if you do the right things.

- Make sure you get plenty of calcium, vitamin D, and physical activity.
- Maintain a healthy weight, limit your alcohol intake, and don't smoke.
- Talk to your doctor about detecting bone disease and medications to treat it. Discuss also the effect of other illnesses and medicines you are already taking.
- Practice fall prevention. Take steps to maintain your vision and balance, eliminate trip hazards, install handrails and grab bars, and wear supportive, rubber-soled shoes.

The problem is absorption

Vitamin B12 is found naturally in animal foods, including meat, fish, poultry, eggs, and milk, as well as fortified breakfast cereals.

Unfortunately, some people don't absorb B12 very well. Stabler says a vitamin B12 deficiency is common in five to 10 percent of people over age 60. One reason is older people don't have enough stomach acid to release the vitamin from the protein in foods.

"A person cannot tell if they are getting enough B12 on a usual diet since it is a stomach failure to absorb that causes the problem," she advises. If you think you might be having problems, talk with your doctor about having your B12 and homocysteine levels checked.

Back brace for back pain

★★☆

Relieve pressure with new designs

Forget those old, stiff, heavy back braces. It's the 21st century, and braces have been re-engineered to offer you more flexibility in a lightweight design. Instead of keeping you from moving, they take the pressure off your back and let you move around freely.

How it works

Roughly 80 percent of back pain is caused by muscle strain, arthritis, or a degenerated, bulging or displaced disc. Most people recover within four to six weeks of an episode of back pain. However, if your problem continues, your doctor may prescribe a back brace to help ease your pain.

Although back braces have been around for several decades, the old designs restricted your movements by immobilizing your back. They also caused other problems such as weak abdominal muscles. The current crop of redesigned braces are cool, comfortable, and made from lightweight breathable materials.

These new braces provide relief from back pain by unloading pressure from your discs and shifting the pressure to your stomach muscles or hips. Certain braces actually lift the load off your discs by separating them. They also may help relieve chronic pain that radiates down your leg.

Lighten your back's load

In a recent clinical study, this type of "pneumatic" brace was shown to be highly effective when compared to a non-pneumatic brace in people with radiating leg pain from disc problems.

After 12 weeks, both groups reported less back and leg pain, but those using the pneumatic brace felt significantly less back pain and an even greater improvement in their legs. Their ability to carry out daily activities improved to a greater extent, as did their flexibility and emotional health.

Not a cure-all

The idea behind a back brace is not to cure your pain but to relieve it temporarily so you can continue your daily activities. The brace helps interrupt pain signals to your brain, giving you time to strengthen your back through physical therapy and exercise.

You should not wear a pneumatic brace more than a few hours at a time or you may further weaken your abdominal muscles. You can lower your risk by exercising to strengthen your lower stomach muscles.

Wearing a back brace does not give you a license to do anything you want. You may feel better, but remember to be careful when performing any demanding activities.

Try less caffeine for less pain

In a research project in Vermont, people who complained of back pain said they drank an average of three 8-ounce cups of coffee a day — that's a whopping 400 milligrams (mg) of caffeine. People without back pain drank half that amount. If you would like to cut back on caffeine, here are some sources to avoid.

Food, beverage, or medicine	Serving size	Caffeine content
Excedrin, Extra strength	2 tablets	130 mg
Midol	2 tablets	120 mg
Anacin, Regular strength	2 tablets	64 mg
Mountain Dew	12 ozs	54 mg
Diet Coke	12 ozs	46 mg
Dr. Pepper	12 oz	41 mg
Sunkist Orange Soda	12 ozs	40 mg
Chocolate ice cream	1 cup	4 mg
Pepsi	12 oz	38 mg
Diet lemon-flavored instant iced tea	8 ozs	36 mg
Tea, brewed 3 minutes	6 ozs	36 mg
Coca-Cola Classic	12 oz	34 mg
Hershey's dark chocolate bar	1.5 oz	31 mg
Nestea with lemon and sweetener	12 oz	16 mg
Hershey's milk chocolate bar	1.5 oz	10 mg

Beta blockers for essential tremor

★★☆

Surprising help for shaky hands

For millions of movie fans, ET was a cute alien who wanted to phone home. But for millions of older adults, ET is a nuisance they wish would go away.

Essential tremor, or ET, is a neurological disorder similar to Parkinson's disease. As many as one in five people older than 65 may have this condition.

With essential tremor, your hands tremble, usually while in use. This means you may have difficulty eating or writing. Your head, neck, arms, and voice may also tremble. While more annoying and embarrassing than dangerous, essential tremor causes its share of problems.

Beta blockers, prescription drugs used to treat high blood pressure, may provide relief for this condition.

How it works

The cause of essential tremor is unknown, but new research shows the part of the brain called the cerebellum does not appear to function correctly in people with this condition. The cerebellum coordinates muscle movement so any problem here could result in irregular movements in different parts of your body.

Medications seem to help improve symptoms in most patients. Along with anti-seizure drugs, beta-blockers are the first line of therapy to treat this condition. These drugs work by blocking the action of substances called neurotransmitters that are released when neurons are stimulated. They particularly work on compounds related to adrenaline. By blocking these rapid-firing neurotransmitters, the drugs help your muscles experience fewer erratic movements.

Success for 60 percent

The beta blocker propranolol has long been one of the standard treatments for essential tremor. It helps about 60 percent of people with ET and is especially effective for shaky hands.

Two recent studies shed more light on treating ET with beta blockers.

- A South Korean study compared propranolol with arotinolol, another beta blocker, and found that arotinolol may be just as effective. People in the study showed similar improvement in daily tasks, such as eating, drinking, and dressing, as well as writing and water pouring.

- A Bulgarian study examined the differences between propranolol and primidone, an anti-seizure medication often used to treat ET. Primidone worked better for kinetic tremors, or those occurring during movement,

---

Quiet the quakes of ET

There are several things you can do to reduce the impact essential tremor has on your life.
- Learn as much as you can about your condition.
- Avoid stressful situations.
- Talk to your doctor about any medications you're taking that may make your tremors worse.
- Try massage therapy.
- Learn some relaxation techniques, like deep breathing, meditation, hypnosis, or biofeedback.
- Avoid caffeine.
- Ask your doctor about Botulinum toxin injections.
- Discuss acupuncture as an alternate therapy.
- Alcohol may temporarily reduce tremors, but is not considered an appropriate treatment.
- Consider surgery if you have an extreme case of ET.

---

while propranolol worked better for postural tremors, or those caused by being in a certain position.

No treatment, including beta blockers, is a cure for ET. But propranolol or primidone — or the combination — may help lessen the severity of the tremors and improve your ability to function.

Beware of side effects

You need a prescription for beta blockers. Follow the directions exactly. The usual dosage of propranolol is 40 mg twice a day, although your doctor may increase it up to 320 mg per day. In the South Korean study, people received 10 to 30 mg of arotinolol twice a day. To be safe, tell your doctor about any other conditions you have and which other medications you're taking.

You should be aware of some potential side effects with beta blockers. These include diarrhea, upset stomach, slow heartbeat, headache, dizziness, drowsiness, trouble sleeping, decreased sexual ability, skin rash, itching, loss of appetite, stuffy nose, and shortness of breath.

Remember, medication doesn't help everyone with essential tremor. But if you're one of the lucky ones, you can regain control of your movements — and your life.

Blue-green algae for fatigue

Energize with foods — not supplements

Feeling tired and run down? Thinking about following the advice of those ads that tell you blue-green algae pills will pep you up? Well, there's an outside chance they might help. But don't count on it.

How it works

Blue-green algae — commonly thought of as pond scum — are microscopic plants that are among Earth's most primitive life forms. Their deep blue-green color comes from pigments such as chlorophyll, phycocyanin, and carotenoids.

Edible blue-green algae are rich in nutrients and have been used for food for thousands of years. Today, algae supplements are touted as miracle workers that can do everything from boost your energy and brighten your mood to help you lose weight.

Spirulina is one form of blue-green algae sold as a health supplement. Promoters of spirulina as a health food claim this microscopic plant contains 60 percent protein, all the essential amino acids, many phytochemicals, the essential fatty acid gammalinolenic acid (GLA), plus many others.

They also claim it's the world's best source of vitamin B12, one reason they believe it can help you beat fatigue. Vitamin B12 works with another B vitamin, folic acid, to help you build healthy red blood cells. If you're low in B12, you can experience fatigue, among other symptoms. So replenishing your B12 levels could help increase your energy.

Spirulina is also rich in easily absorbable iron, another important red blood cell ingredient.

Watch out for contamination

The nutritional content of blue-green algae depends on the location and environment where it is grown. Experts are concerned about the quality of blue-green algae harvested in the wild.

One example involves an algae supplement taken from Upper Klamath Lake in southern Oregon. Officials found that a toxic variety of algae had made lake waters unsafe for drinking or bathing. They then realized an even greater danger came from eating the health food products harvested from the lake.

Most blue-green algae products are obtained from lakes like Upper Klamath all over the world. There is no way to know what kind of unhealthy material — from heavy metals to animal feces — is also collected from these lakes.

Is spirulina safe?

Producers of spirulina point out it is grown in a controlled environment that keeps out pollutants. However, it also is sold as a dietary supplement, which means manufacturers don't have to prove to the U.S. Food and Drug Administration (FDA) or anyone else that the product is safe. The FDA must prove it is not safe before it can take any action.

> Don't let low energy bring you down. Stay active and full of zip with a balanced, vitamin-rich diet, moderate exercise, and enough deep, restful sleep.

People who use spirulina may believe they reap many benefits, but these claims are unproven. Studies have been done on animals and in the laboratory, but it is still unknown whether spirulina interacts with drugs or causes any long-term chronic problems.

As the FDA points out, all the nutrients in spirulina are readily available from food — and at a much lower cost. You're better off enjoying the nutritional benefits of whole foods than taking your chances with pond scum.

Botox for BPH

Wrinkle remedy helps prostate

Botox (*botulinum toxin A*) is usually thought of as something used mostly by women to smooth out wrinkles. But here's a purpose for men only — reducing the problems of an enlarged prostate gland.

Benign prostatic hyperplasia (BPH) is a condition where the prostate becomes enlarged and puts pressure on the urethra. Although it's not life threatening, it does cause unpleasant urinary symptoms and can lead to more serious problems down the road.

The prostate gland has two types of cells — glandular and smooth muscle. Medical treatment for BPH focuses either on shrinking the glandular cells or relaxing the smooth muscle tissue. There are also a number of surgical options.

Unfortunately, treatment options all have some sort of downside, ranging from dizziness to incontinence to various degrees of sexual distress. Men with BPH generally have to choose between the lesser of evils.

How it works

Botulinum toxin A — produced by the bacterium *Clostridium botulinum* — contains the same toxin that causes food poisoning. It blocks the release of acetylcholine, a nerve-cell chemical that tells muscles to contract. Large doses, such as in botulism poisoning, can shut down your entire system. The small doses used for cosmetic procedures simply keep facial muscles from contracting, resulting in fewer wrinkles and smoother skin.

Now Botox is being looked at as a possible treatment for urological problems, particularly BPH. Other types of injections have been used to treat this problem, and they appear to work by killing tissue cells and shrinking the prostate gland back to normal. Botox may work by relaxing the smooth muscle in the prostate.

Initial research is promising

Using Botox to treat BPH is only experimental so far, but a few small studies have had good results. A team from the University of Pittsburgh School of Medicine and Chang Gung Memorial Hospital in Taiwan gave Botox injections to 11 men aged 50 to 82 who had BPH symptoms. Those symptoms were reduced 62 percent compared to a placebo. The men's quality of life scores rose 56 percent, urinary flow increased significantly, and they reported no significant side effects.

> BPH affects about half the men between 51 and 60 years old, jumping to 90 percent for those over 80. Some men may not have symptoms, and treatment is necessary only when it becomes bothersome. Between 20 and 30 percent of men will require treatment by age 80.

Another study, at the University Hospital Agostino Gemelli in Rome, had similar results. Doctors there injected 30 men with either Botox or saline solution. Symptoms did not change in the control group, but after two months, the Botox group had a 65 percent improvement in urinary symptoms. No serious side effects were reported from either group.

Both studies concluded that Botox is a promising alternative treatment for BPH, but more research is needed. The U.S. Food and Drug Administration currently has approved Botox for only a few specific uses.

Get your doctor's advice

Although BPH is not life threatening, its symptoms can lead to serious complications. It can prevent the bladder from emptying completely, which in turn causes infections and incontinence. Some symptoms of BPH are also similar to those for prostate cancer, so it's important to see a doctor for a thorough diagnosis.

Drug side effects and aversion to surgery sometimes prompt men to avoid treatment for BPH. Researchers are optimistic that Botox injections can become a more acceptable treatment option in the future.

Broccoli sprouts for ulcers

Killer veggie destroys *H. pylori*

Former President George H. Bush might not be a fan of broccoli, but he might be impressed with broccoli sprouts. These tasty sprouts could rid your stomach of *H. pylori*, bacteria that can cause ulcers.

How it works

Some strains of *H. pylori*, or *Helicobacter pylori*, are strong enough to survive a battle with antibiotics. But they may not be able to escape from broccoli sprouts and their powerful disease-fighter sulforaphane. In test-tube studies, this natural plant compound wiped out the toughest *H. pylori* bacteria, even those resistant to regular antibiotics.

Sulforaphane apparently acts as a natural antibiotic, although how it does this is not clearly understood. But studies show it has the powerful ability to kill *H. pylori* not only outside the cells, but inside, where regular antibiotics cannot reach. *H. pylori* often hide in cells lining your stomach, making it difficult to cure the infection. By eating broccoli sprouts with this mighty phytochemical, you may knock out your ulcer once and for all.

Sprouts wipe out *H. pylori*

H. pylori infection is a major health problem throughout the world, and in addition to ulcers, it's associated with stomach cancer. Researchers think broccoli sprouts also boost production of anti-cancer enzymes.

According to a preliminary study, broccoli sprouts' ability to destroy *H. pylori* shows promise. Researchers enlisted the help of nine people who tested positive for *H. pylori*.

These study participants, who were divided into three groups, ate 14, 28, or 56 grams of broccoli sprouts twice a day for seven days. On day eight, researchers tested them for the bacteria. Seven of the nine people showed no signs of *H. pylori*. Researchers checked them again on day 35, and six out of the nine were still negative.

More studies need to be done to determine the most efficient dose and the proper number of days needed to destroy the

Escape the pain of ulcers

Nonsteroidal anti-inflammatory drugs (NSAIDs) do wonders for pain, but use them with caution. NSAIDs and acetaminophen shut down the enzymes that guard your stomach lining and increase your odds of getting ulcers.

Talk to your doctor about using a safe herbal remedy for pain — and follow these tips to prevent ulcer flare-ups.

- Eat fiber-rich and nutrient-packed foods, like fruits, vegetables, and whole grains. Make sure to get plenty of vitamin C. New research suggests a link between low blood levels of vitamin C and ulcers.
- Space your meals regularly throughout the day instead of having snacks.
- Get a good night's sleep.
- Exercise regularly.
- Stop smoking.
- Manage your stress with a hobby or yoga classes.
- Cut down on coffee and alcohol.

bacteria. A higher dose than the one used in the study could be even more effective. In addition, the study period was only seven days, whereas the proper regiment of an antibiotic is 10 to 14 days.

Crunch into good health

Fresh sprouts have gotten a lot of bad press lately, but if you miss that healthy crunch on your favorite sandwich, reach for broccoli sprouts.

Developed by researchers at Johns Hopkins University School of Medicine, these powerful veggies are also a good source of fiber, vitamin C, and calcium.

Broccoli sprouts are cruciferous vegetables that belong to the brassica plant family. Broccoli, cauliflower, cabbage, brussels sprouts, and turnips are also members.

Researchers think chewing these vegetables uncooked unleashes glucosinolates, the compound needed to make sulforaphane. Broccoli sprouts are very rich in glucosinolates. In fact, they contain from 20 to 50 times more of this compound than regular broccoli.

Broccoli sprouts are not sold at every grocery store, so you might have to search your area to find one that sells them.

Calcium for colon cancer

★★☆

Bone-builder fights polyps

Most women know one of the best ways to fight osteoporosis is to get enough calcium. But better bones isn't the only thing calcium will do for you. It also helps keep colon cancer — the second-leading killer cancer — at bay.

Numerous studies have shown that calcium is associated with a modestly reduced risk of colorectal cancer — cancer of the colon or rectum. Since colon cancer is so common, even a small reduction in risk can prevent many cancer cases.

The greatest risk factors for colorectal cancer include age, genetics, and a history of polyps — small growths that can develop into cancer — in the colon. Your best defense against this deadly disease is regular screening and a diet that skimps on fat and loads up on fiber. After you've done that, help keep your colon healthy by making sure you get enough calcium.

How it works

Calcium cannot slow the growth of cancer, but this important mineral may help treat or prevent precancerous changes, such as polyps, in your colon. Researchers think calcium may help reduce your risk of colorectal cancer by binding bile acids and ionized fatty acids, which keeps them from interacting with and irritating the colon lining.

Pick the right calcium for you		
Form of calcium	**Calcium percentage**	**Pros and cons**
Calcium carbonate	40 percent calcium	Economical, difficult to absorb so must be taken with food
Calcium citrate	24 percent calcium	More expensive, easier to absorb
Calcium gluconate	9 percent calcium	Most expensive, difficult to break down

Calcium also may prevent overgrowth of the cells lining the intestinal tract by regulating cell responses and signaling. Another theory is that calcium helps block cancer-causing agents from attacking the lining of the colon.

Recent studies show positive results

Up until 1998, researchers weren't convinced there was any relationship between calcium and colorectal polyps. Since then, however, the evidence has mounted.

An American Cancer Society study of more than 126,000 men and women concluded that calcium modestly reduces the risk of colorectal cancer.

A year later, the National Cancer Institute came out with a study of more than 38,000 people saying a high calcium intake, especially from supplements, is associated with fewer polyps in the colon.

Unfortunately, results from another study showed that very high calcium intakes, above the recommended amount, could increase a man's risk of prostate cancer. The challenge for researchers is how to balance the impact of calcium on osteoporosis, colon cancer, and prostate cancer.

Where to get calcium

Dairy products are the main food source of calcium. In this case, however, that may not be the best place to get your colon cancer protection. Dairy products don't seem to reduce colon cancer risk.

To prevent colon cancer, calcium from supplements — rather than food — seems to be best. But more is not better. The adequate intake (AI) for folks over age 50 is 1,200 milligrams (mg), but colon cancer risk starts decreasing at about 700 mg a day. There's no further improvement above 1,000 mg.

Other foods that provide calcium are leafy green vegetables, especially Chinese cabbage, kale, and broccoli. Grain products have some calcium, and there are a number of calcium-fortified foods, like fruit drinks, juices, and cereals.

The two main choices for supplemental calcium are calcium carbonate and calcium citrate. Many antacids are made from calcium carbonate. See *Tums for osteoporosis* on page 295 to get more details on this handy, inexpensive source of calcium.

Stand firm against colon cancer

The older you are, the higher your risk of developing colon cancer. Do everything you can — starting today — to protect yourself from this deadly disease.

- Eat a high-fiber, low-fat diet.
- Drink plenty of water every day.
- Stop smoking.
- Exercise 30 to 60 minutes a day.
- Ask your doctor about aspirin therapy.
- Avoid red meat and processed meats.
- Cook with olive oil whenever possible.
- Limit alcohol.
- Try some curry dishes.
- Maintain a healthy weight.
- Get regular colon cancer screenings.

Capsaicin cream for arthritis pain

Sidestep side effects with peppers

Send your arthritis pain packing with the power of hot peppers. Over-the-counter pain relief creams containing capsaicin, an ingredient derived from hot peppers, can relieve your aching joints without serious side effects.

How it works

Capsaicin works by depleting substance P, a protein-like compound that transmits pain impulses to your brain. It also releases enzymes that can cause inflammation in your joints.

By reducing the amount of substance P, capsaicin blocks pain signals to your brain by decreasing nerve cell sensitivity. Your pain might still exist, but your brain doesn't know it, so you don't feel it. What's more, capsaicin doesn't cause numbness or other serious side effects like other pain relief medicines.

Pain reduced significantly

In a recent study, researchers tested capsaicin's effect on 36 arthritis sufferers for 42 days. The study participants continued their regular drug and exercise treatments but, in addition, applied capsaicin cream or a placebo (inactive substance) to their hands or knees.

The capsaicin users reported a 38-percent decrease in pain and a

Although products like BenGay and Icy Hot are not effective on chronic pain, they may relieve occasional, mild muscle aches. These products, known as counterirritants, work by stimulating your hot and cold sensory receptors to mask the pain. However, they also leave behind a medicinal odor and require frequent applications.

35-percent improvement in joint stiffness, while the placebo users had very little improvement in pain and stiffness. The study noted that trials of NSAIDs (nonsteroidal anti-inflammatory drugs), like aspirin and ibuprofen, had a 30-percent decrease in pain and a 15-percent improvement in joint stiffness. The researchers concluded that capsaicin was as effective as NSAIDs without serious side effects, like stomach and intestinal bleeding.

Watch out for the burn

Capsaicin reduces arthritis pain in the joints nearest your skin. It can cause a warm, stinging, or burning sensation. But regular use will cause the sensation to fade within a few days. Here are a few other precautions.

---

10 natural solutions to arthritis pain

Some over-the-counter medications can have serious side effects. Help yourself with these natural ways to relieve pain and inflammation, reduce damage to your joints, and ease your morning stiffness.

1 • Eat more vitamin-C-rich foods like oranges and strawberries.
2 • Serve up some delicious cherries. These scarlet fruits can ease your pain better than ibuprofen, with no stomach upset or other side effects.
3 • Add fish to your dinner menu several times a week.
4 • Try primrose oil.
5 • Enjoy foods containing beta-carotene, like carrots, broccoli, and sweet potatoes.
6 • Enhance homemade breads and desserts with flaxseed.
7 • Chop up ginger, and stir it into stew or toss it in your salad.
8 • Try the herb boswellia, known as frankincense in biblical days.
9 • Lubricate your joints with a minimum of six full glasses of water each day.
10 • Mix 2 teaspoons each of apple-cider vinegar and honey in a glass of water, and drink with meals.

- Wash your hands before touching your eyes or contacts. If capsaicin gets in your eyes, flush them with water.

- Don't soak affected area in water or wrap in tight bandages.

- Avoid using on wounds or irritated skin.

- Check with your doctor if you are using other medication or have allergies.

Applying capsaicin to your aching back may give you fast, soothing relief. But some people don't feel pain relief for the first week or two. Nevertheless, persistent use — at least three or four times a day for several weeks — continues to reduce substance P and your feeling of pain.

Capsaicin products, in cream, roll-on, and stick forms, are available in over-the-counter strengths of .025 to .1 percent. Recent clinical trials were split on the concentrations used. Arthritis studies used .025 or .050 percent capsaicin, while nerve disorder studies used .075 percent. Experiment to find the capsaicin strength that works best for you.

> Use your fingers to rub a small amount onto the affected area and massage it in thoroughly three or four times daily. If you're applying the cream to your hands, don't wash it off for at least 30 minutes.

X

You can buy capsaicin products at most drugstores and discount department stores.

Chelation therapy for atherosclerosis

Slam door on sham treatment

It sounds like a marvelous medical magic trick. Just receive a series of injections and — poof! — atherosclerosis disappears. But chelation therapy, like all magicians, is ultimately nothing but a lot of hocus-pocus.

How it works

Chelation therapy involves putting the chemical ethylenedi-amine tetra-acetic acid (EDTA) into your bloodstream, along with several other substances. This treatment has been found to effectively remove toxic metals, like mercury, lead, and cadmium from your blood.

Atherosclerosis is a narrowing and thickening of your arteries due to a buildup of choles-terol-rich plaque. This plaque blocks your blood flow, increasing your risk of heart attack and stroke.

Because of this, some scientists theorized that it could remove calcium deposits on the walls of your arteries, which would help soften hardened arteries and allow blood to flow more freely.

After this theory was disproved, other ideas were proposed, including the most recent that EDTA blocks the creation of free radicals involved in the progression of atherosclerosis. Studies have shown that oxidative stress, which creates those unstable molecules, harms the cells that line the arteries.

Some scientists have suggested that the antioxidant effect of EDTA, together with vitamins and minerals, might hinder this process. But research has not supported the use of chelation therapy for artery disease.

No benefit found

In spite of its lofty claims, chelation therapy does not fare well in scientific studies.

- A recent Canadian study showed chelation therapy with EDTA, vitamins, and minerals provided no additional benefit for people with coronary artery disease who were being treated with proven therapies.

- Another recent Canadian study of 84 people with coronary artery disease showed chelation therapy did not help above the placebo effect.

- A small German study from 1987 determined chelation therapy had no effect on blood flow and was no help to diseased arteries.

Look for more conclusive results in a few years. The National Heart, Lung, and Blood Institute has launched a large-scale, five-year study called Trial to Assess Chelation Therapy, or TACT.

In the meantime, the Federal Trade Commission ordered the American College for Advancement in Medicine, the main promoters of chelation therapy, to stop making false claims about the treatment.

Avoid high costs, health risks

Proponents of chelation therapy say you usually need about 30 treatments. But the amount of treatments ranges from 20 all the way up to 100. Periodic follow-up is also recommended.

This could become expensive, as each treatment costs between $75 and $125. To make matters worse, chelation therapy is rarely covered by health insurance.

Besides its steep monetary cost, chelation therapy may take its toll on your health. Possible side effects include irregular heartbeat, kidney damage, bleeding, blood clots, skin problems, low blood sugar, and allergic reactions to EDTA.

It's best to stay away from this treatment. Stick to effective approaches to fight atherosclerosis, like a heart-healthy diet, regular exercise, and proven treatments to lower your blood pressure and cholesterol levels.

Chiropractic for back pain

★★☆

Find relief with alternative treatment

Many people have found relief for their back pain through chiropractic care. And at least one study shows chiropractic may work slightly better than physical therapy. So if nothing else seems to relieve your constant ache, you may want to consider this alternative form of medicine.

How it works

The focus of chiropractic care involves your nervous system and spine. Your spine provides two functions. It allows you to move freely, and it holds and protects your spinal cord. You have 33 bony vertebrae in your spinal column. Hundreds of nerves branch off the spine through openings in the vertebrae.

Chiropractors believe tiny misalignments in the vertebrae, called subluxations, can pinch these nerves. When this happens, your body parts served by the nerves can't function correctly. By adjusting your vertebrae and eliminating the subluxations, chiropractors relieve the pressure on your nerves and allow your body to heal.

Support for chiropractic care

A study at the University of California at Los Angeles compared the effectiveness of medical and chiropractic care in low back pain sufferers. The study followed 681 people for a six-month period. They were randomly assigned to one of four groups.

- Medical care only. Subjects received back care instructions, medications, and flexibility and strengthening exercises.

- Medical care with physical therapy. Subjects received the above medical care plus one or more of the following: heat or cold therapy, ultrasound, electrical muscle stimulation, soft-tissue and joint mobilization, therapeutic exercise, and traction.

- Chiropractic care only. Subjects received spinal manipulation plus back care instructions and flexibility and strengthening exercises.

- Chiropractic care with other therapy. Subjects received the above chiropractic care plus one or more of the following: heat therapy, ultrasound, and electrical muscle stimulation.

The difference between the groups was clinically insignificant. However, chiropractic care with additional therapy appeared to work slightly better than medical care with physical therapy.

Watch out for quacks

Some chiropractors believe improperly aligned vertebrae create blockages of nerve energy that cause illness. They claim spinal manipulation can cure everything from asthma to diabetes. However, scientific evidence does not support these ideas. Some chiropractors are even expanding into "holistic" healing, giving advice on nutrition, herbs, and other alternative remedies.

Another group has rejected their original chiropractic teachings and limit their focus to musculoskeletal problems. Working with science, they show how manipulation can relieve neck and back problems, just like physical therapy. These chiropractors are members of the National Association for Chiropractic Medicine.

Because you have so many choices, you'll want to check credentials carefully before committing to any chiropractor. Call your state's Chiropractic Board of Examiners before you make an appointment. Look in your telephone book under state government for the number, or go online to the National Board of Chiropractic Examiners at *www.nbce.org*, where you'll find links to the state organizations. They can tell you if the chiropractor is licensed and whether he has any complaints against him.

Before trying a chiropractor, see your doctor for a diagnosis of your problem first. Some studies have described cases of stroke occurring from small artery tears after neck manipulation. However, it's not clear if the treatment caused the strokes or if the people involved already had damaged neck arteries. It's best to have your own doctor check you out thoroughly before trying an alternative treatment.

Break your bad habits

You can prevent future back attacks and ease lower back pain with these natural remedies.

- Exercise for at least 30 minutes three or four times a week. Stretch before and after you exercise. Include exercises that strengthen your lower abdominal muscles, which help support your back.
- Lose the potbelly. It's especially hard on your back. Your back muscles exert 50 pounds of force to balance a 10-pound potbelly.
- Stop smoking. Doctors aren't sure why, but smoking aggravates back problems.
- Don't sleep on your stomach. Sleep on a firm mattress with a pillow under your knees if you sleep on your back. Put it between your knees if you sleep on your side.
- Lift heavy objects properly. Squat down, keeping your back straight. Hold the object close to your body, and use your arms and legs, rather than your back, to lift the weight.

Chiropractic can be a safe, natural alternative to drugs or surgery for back pain. Just remember to use caution when considering chiropractic care, and don't hesitate to ask questions.

Chitosan for weight loss

Steer clear of 'fat magnet'

Perhaps you've heard the enticing claims about the weight loss supplement chitosan. Eat all you want. Lose weight without dieting. Block fat, trap fat, zap fat. It all sounds too good to be true. That's because it is.

How it works
Chitosan is a fiber supplement made from chitin, a substance found in the shells of shrimp, lobster, and crabs.

People who sell chitosan claim it binds with fat and shuttles the fat out of your body so you absorb less of it. But in practice, that's a fish story.

Helps only slightly — if at all
Scientists who studied chitosan's effect on weight discovered the facts don't measure up to the hype.

- A small English study found that chitosan, by itself, doesn't work. People in the study took 2 grams of chitosan a day but made no other changes to their diet. After four weeks, they did not show any significant difference in weight.

- In a study of 69 mildly obese women, those taking 3 grams of chitosan a day lost an average of only 2.2 pounds after eight weeks of treatment.

- A University of California-Davis study measured fecal fat in an attempt to gauge chitosan's success. Although 15 men took 4.5 grams of chitosan a day, they showed only a slight increase in fecal fat when using chitosan. The amount of fat trapped, about 1.1 grams or 9.9 calories a day, is not enough to have any meaningful effect on weight loss.

- Japanese researchers determined chitosan does have a mild cholesterol-lowering effect — but no effect on weight loss.

Rate your weight

The body mass index (BMI) chart will help you decide if your weight is in a healthy range. A BMI of 25 or below is considered healthy. A BMI above 25 generally means you are overweight and over 30 indicates you are obese.

Weight	130	140	150	160	170	180	190	200
Height								
5'0"	25	27	29	31	33	35	37	39
5'1"	25	26	28	30	32	34	36	38
5'2"	24	26	27	29	31	33	35	37
5'3"	23	25	27	28	30	32	34	35
5'4"	22	24	26	27	29	31	33	34
5'5"	22	23	25	27	28	30	32	33
5'6"	21	23	24	26	27	29	31	32
5'7"	20	22	23	25	27	28	30	31
5'8"	20	21	23	24	26	27	29	30
5'9"	19	21	22	24	25	27	28	30
5'10"	19	20	22	23	24	26	27	29
5'11"	18	20	21	22	24	25	26	28
6'0"	18	19	20	22	23	24	26	27
6'1"	17	18	20	21	22	24	25	26
6'2"	17	18	19	21	22	23	24	26
6'3"	16	17	19	20	21	22	24	25

Avoid allergies and other pitfalls

How much chitosan is recommended if you're trying to lose weight? Recommendations range from 1 to 5 grams a day. If you take it in the form of 500-milligram capsules, that would be a total of two to 10 capsules a day spread out during mealtimes.

Unfortunately, with chitosan you have more to worry about than how much to take or whether you're wasting your money.

Beware of chitosan if you're allergic to shellfish. Pregnant or nursing women and young children should also avoid chitosan. That's because of the chance of contamination with heavy metals, such as lead, mercury, iron, and copper.

Experts suspect that long-term use of chitosan may make it difficult for your body to absorb key minerals, like calcium, magnesium, and selenium, as well as vitamins A, D, E, and K. Other side effects include nausea, diarrhea, gas, and constipation.

Instead of popping chitosan pills, stick to tried-and-true weight loss methods. These include eating a healthy diet that's low in fat and high in fiber and exercising regularly.

Remember, the only surefire way to lose weight is to burn more calories than you take in. Relying on chitosan supplements to help you "zap" fat will probably just make you crabby.

Chocolate for heart disease

Toast your health with cocoa

A steaming mug of hot cocoa or a luxurious dark chocolate bar may sound decadent, but these tempting treats just might help you fight heart disease.

How it works

You may be surprised to discover that chocolate is a plant food. Chocolate is processed from the cocoa bean found in the fruit pod of the cacao tree, says Mary Engler, Ph.D., a School of Nursing professor and vascular physiologist at the University of California at San Francisco. Dark chocolate gets its heart-healthy benefits mainly from antioxidant flavonoids like catechin and epicatechin.

Studies suggest flavonoid-rich dark chocolate or cocoa powder may help cut heart disease risk in these ways.

- increases blood flow

- lowers blood pressure

- thwarts free radical damage to LDL cholesterol to help prevent clogged arteries

- inhibits blood clots

- diminishes inflammation

- improves arteries' flexibility and dilating ability

Besides, clinical studies suggest that chocolate does not raise cholesterol. "The fat in chocolate (cocoa butter) contains approximately 35 percent oleic acid — the monounsaturated fat found in olive oil — and 60 percent saturated fat, which is 35 percent stearic acid and 25 percent palmitic acid," says Engler. Scientists think the cholesterol-raising effects of palmitic acid may be offset by stearic and oleic acid.

Dark chocolate even provides magnesium, copper, and potassium.

Plain cocoa powder has a shelf life of one year once you've opened the container. But unopened cocoa powder can be stored indefinitely. Cocoa mixes only last about eight months.

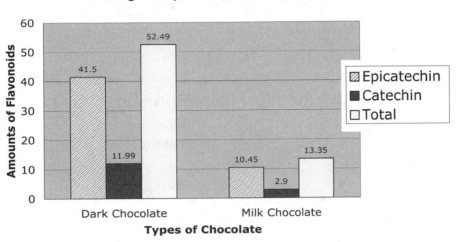

Flavonoids in Chocolate
Per 100 grams (3 to 3 1/2 ounces) of chocolat

Stay tuned for stronger evidence

A review of the research on chocolate and cocoa verified that antioxidants in chocolate flavonoids may help prevent free radical damage. What's more, these exciting studies have appeared since the review.

- Researchers comparing the antioxidant content of cocoa, tea, and red wine were surprised to find that cocoa has the highest levels.

- A two-week study of 21 adults found that a daily serving of high-flavonoid dark chocolate helped improve blood vessels' ability to expand.

- A study of 13 adults with mild high blood pressure suggested that a daily dose of dark chocolate may help lower blood pressure slightly after a few weeks.

- A British study found that dark chocolate may help prevent platelets from clumping into blood clots, but milk chocolate and white chocolate don't have the same effect.

Yet most of these studies are too small or too brief to prove that chocolate works safely for everyone over the long-term. "This field is only at the beginning in terms of the initial positive heart benefits with dark chocolate," says Engler. "Much more research needs to be done."

Sample the new high-flavonoid chocolates

Milk chocolate has fewer nutritious flavonoids than dark chocolate — and white chocolate has nearly none. Even dark chocolates are not all the same.

"Traditional processing conserves only 50 to 75 percent of the total cocoa flavonoids," says Engler. "Dark chocolate should be processed to minimize loss of these important flavonoids. Flavonoid levels in chocolate are preserved approximately 70 to 95 percent when heat and alkalization are reduced during processing."

The milk in milk chocolate bars could prevent your body from absorbing chocolate's flavonoids, according to one small study. But another study — on hot cocoa with milk — disagreed. Perhaps one study measured flavonoids more accurately or maybe the amount of milk is the key. Scientists need more research to unwrap an answer.

Cocoapro, the cocoa in Dove dark chocolate, is specially processed to retain more flavonoids. When buying chocolate, look for the Cocoapro logo. A new Cocoapro product, CocoVia, is available by calling 1-866-262-6266 or going online to *www.cocovia.com*. CocoVia snacks contain cholesterol-fighting phytosterols as well as 100 milligrams of healthy flavonoids.

According to one study, you need around 125 grams — about 4.25 ounces — of flavonoid-rich chocolate daily to get heart-healthy antioxidant benefits. But don't eat more than one or two small bars a day. Chocolate has plenty of fat and calories — and gaining weight is bad for your heart.

To help keep your flavonoid levels from tapering off, Engler suggests eating other foods rich in the same flavonoid as chocolate. Good choices include green and black tea, sweet cherries, apples, purple grapes, blackberries, red wine, and raspberries.

Chromium for diabetes

Trusty mineral tackles blood sugar

Many people have taken a shine to chromium. In fact, it ranks among the most frequently purchased supplements. But before you shell out money for this popular pill, check out the theory behind chromium's success — and the evidence that supports it.

How it works

Chromium is a trace mineral found naturally in plants, animals, and soil. You can also find it in supplement form as chromium picolinate, which is easier for your body to absorb. This is especially handy for people with diabetes who need more chromium but have a harder time converting it to a usable form.

Chromium helps regulate glucose, or blood sugar, by increasing the action of insulin. Experts theorize that chromium teams up with a protein called low molecular weight chromium-binding substance (LMWCr) to kick-start the insulin receptor. In a domino effect, this prompts the cellular signaling mechanism to do its job and let glucose into the cells.

High doses lower blood sugar

Perhaps the strongest evidence for chromium comes from Dr. Richard Anderson's 1997 study that showed chromium picolinate reduced glucose and insulin concentrations in people with type 2 diabetes in China.

Glucose, a simple sugar, gives your body energy. This key carbohydrate can also be stored in your liver and muscles as glycogen until it's needed as fuel. Insulin, a hormone produced by your pancreas, helps control glucose concentrations in your blood. If you don't produce enough insulin, you end up with high blood sugar, or hyperglycemia — a symptom of diabetes.

For four months, the 180 people in the study received either a placebo or chromium picolinate. One supplement group took 200 micrograms (mcg) of chromium picolinate a day, while the other took 1,000 mcg a day.

Both supplement groups significantly decreased their insulin levels and their glycosylated hemoglobin, a sign of high blood sugar. Those in the higher dose group also slashed their glucose levels.

But people in the study weighed an average of only 152 pounds and their dietary intake of chromium before the study was not measured. That might explain why other studies have been inconclusive.

While taking chromium supplements for diabetes seems promising, many health professionals say there is not enough solid evidence to wholeheartedly recommend it.

Proceed with caution

If you choose to supplement your diet with chromium, aim for at least 200 mcg a day. Some experts even recommend taking as much as 1,000 mcg a day.

Keep in mind that this far exceeds the Institute of Medicine's Adequate Intake of 20 mcg a day for women over 50 and 30 mcg a day for men over 50. Although chromium seems safe, there is a lack of information about the long-term effects of chromium supplementation, especially at high doses.

Of some concern is a recent University of Alabama study that found chromium picolinate causes DNA damage in fruit flies. Similar findings have been reported in studies of rats. While this does not necessarily translate into danger for humans, the possibility of danger remains.

Talk with your doctor before taking chromium supplements for diabetes. It might lower the amount of medication you'll need. If you suffer from depression or bipolar disorder, chromium supplements might not be a good idea.

Instead of relying on chromium supplements, make sure to get enough chromium from your diet. Good sources include liver, whole grains, nuts, cheese, broccoli, processed meats, prunes, asparagus, mushrooms, coffee, and tea.

Cinnamon for diabetes

★★☆

Spice slashes blood sugar

A spoonful of sugar helps the medicine go down — but a spoonful of cinnamon does much, much more. Cinnamon is well known as a tasty addition to buns and apple pies. But this popular spice gave diabetes researchers a big surprise when it succeeded in lowering blood sugar just as well as the nutrient they were studying.

How it works

It turns out cinnamon's active ingredient, a polyphenol compound called methylhydroxy chalcone polymer (MHCP), mimics the action of insulin in your body and helps control blood sugar levels.

Cinnamon may work to beat diabetes in other ways, too. Many diabetics have higher blood levels of fats called triglycerides and LDL or "bad" cholesterol. Insulin partly controls these as well as your blood sugar, and studies showed that cinnamon helped lower unhealthy levels of fat and cholesterol.

Diabetics also have a high amount of free radicals circulating in their bodies, and lab experiments showed cinnamon was effective in neutralizing these damaging molecules.

Lowers dangerous fats and cholesterol

The strongest evidence for cinnamon comes from a recent Pakistani study of 30 men and 30 women with diabetes. People in the study took either 1 gram, 3 grams, or 6 grams of cinnamon, in the form of cinnamon capsules, each day for 40 days. Other study participants took equivalent amounts of placebo.

3 more reasons to love cinnamon	
Beats bad bacteria	Lab tests show cinnamon can kill *E. coli*, a dangerous bacteria that can cause severe diarrhea and flu-like symptoms.
Peps up digestion	Scientists aren't sure how it works, but adding some cinnamon to your meals could help relieve frequent indigestion.
Soothes cuts and scrapes	Cinnamon kills bacteria, numbs pain, and stops bleeding. After you wash and dry your cut, shake on some cinnamon powder and cover with a bandage.

People taking cinnamon, regardless of the dose, saw several significant improvements.

- Fasting blood sugar dropped 18 to 29 percent.
- Total cholesterol levels fell 12 to 26 percent, while LDL cholesterol decreased by 7 to 27 percent.
- Triglyceride levels plummeted by 23 to 30 percent.

The positive effects of cinnamon linger. Even 20 days after stopping cinnamon treatment, people often maintained lower blood sugar, cholesterol, and triglyceride levels.

While cinnamon seems extremely promising, more research is needed to support it. Keep your eyes open for future cinnamon studies.

Half-teaspoon does whole lot of good

You don't need mass quantities of cinnamon to reap its benefits. Just 1 gram, or about one-half teaspoon, each day will do the trick. In fact, even smaller amounts probably help.

It's easy to add cinnamon to your diet. Sprinkle some on your oatmeal, cereal, toast, yogurt, apples, and other fruit. You can even use it to spice up your meats and vegetables, such as cooked carrots, winter squash, or sweet potatoes. Swizzle cinnamon sticks in your hot cider, coffee drinks, and juices to add a healthy benefit to your beverages.

Unlike prescription drugs, cinnamon has no side effects to worry about. Even if it doesn't help, it shouldn't hurt. But there are some things to keep in mind.

- Don't eat cinnamon oil. It can be toxic even in small amounts.
- Don't fill up on cinnamon buns, pies, and other high-calorie sweets that contain cinnamon. Just make cinnamon part of a healthy diet.

There might be more proven remedies for diabetes than cinnamon, but you'll be hard-pressed to find a tastier one.

Coffee for diabetes

★★☆

Reduce your risk for type 2

Wake up and smell the coffee. What you drink for breakfast may determine your future health. Start your mornings off right to avoid type 2 diabetes.

If your breakfast includes a steaming mug of java, you're well on your way. This common eye-opener has opened the eyes of quite a few researchers with its uncommon powers.

A few cups a day keeps diabetes away

Long-term studies show that people who drink more than a few cups of coffee every day have a lower risk of developing type 2 diabetes. Research conducted in different countries yielded similar results.

- Men who drank six or more cups of coffee a day slashed their risk by more than 50 percent in a recent Harvard study. Women who drank four to six cups cut their risk by 30 percent.

- Swedish women who drank five to six cups a day lowered their risk by more than 60 percent.

- People who drank a whopping 10 cups or more a day benefited the most in a Finnish study. Women reduced their risk by 80 percent, while men lowered their risk by more than 50 percent.

All of the above studies relied on questionnaires from the participants, so a direct cause-and-effect link could not be established. But the evidence remains very strong.

Strong — but not unanimous. For example, the National Institute of Diabetes and Digestive and Kidney Diseases found no link between coffee drinking and the risk of type 2 diabetes.

How it works

Just as you might appreciate coffee for different reasons — the aroma, the taste, that jolt of caffeine — scientists have different theories about what makes coffee tick.

They know caffeine hampers your body's ability to control blood sugar in the short term. That's why some researchers strongly advise people with diabetes to avoid it (see *'Grounds' for concern* on page 112). However, caffeine may actually help over the long haul as your tolerance for it builds.

But coffee's real hero might not be caffeine at all. That honor could belong to chlorogenic acid, which helps regulate blood sugar.

Coffee's high levels of antioxidants, mostly in the form of chlorogenic acid, may also improve insulin sensitivity by protecting your cells from damage.

Other ingredients, including magnesium, potassium, and niacin, could also play key roles in staving off diabetes.

Get the scoop on coffee

Keep the following tips in mind before filling your mug.

- Consider decaffeinated coffee, which still has chlorogenic acids but very little of the caffeine of regular coffee. Go easy on the sugar, too.

- Stick with filtered coffee. Boiled coffee, the kind you get with a French press coffee maker, might not provide the same benefits.

- Use common sense. Don't go overboard and substitute mass quantities of coffee for a healthy diet, exercise, weight loss, and other proven strategies to prevent diabetes.

You can enjoy a cup of coffee just about anywhere — including your favorite bookstore. When buying coffee to brew at home, buy only enough for a week, and store it in a cool, dark place to keep it fresh.

Taking a few coffee breaks throughout the day just might give you a break from diabetes later.

'Grounds' for concern

If you already have diabetes, trouble might be brewing along with your coffee.

Researchers from Duke University measured the effects of caffeine on 14 coffee drinkers with type 2 diabetes.

Caffeine didn't make much of an impact on an empty stomach. But when these people had caffeine with their meals, their glucose levels shot up 21 percent and their insulin levels skyrocketed 48 percent.

Because of these surprising results, the researchers recommend cutting back on caffeine or even eliminating it from your diet entirely.

Keep in mind the study was very small and used caffeine pills rather than coffee. Even so, it's probably wise to drink coffee in moderation.

Copper bracelet for rheumatoid arthritis

$2 billion down the drain

Ancient Egyptians had a stylish cure for arthritis — copper jewelry. Even today, many people claim wearing a piece of copper against your skin allows your body to absorb this essential mineral and relieve arthritis symptoms.

How it works

Some experts say it's possible that a copper deficiency contributes to rheumatoid arthritis, although there's no proof that wearing copper jewelry helps increase your body's mineral levels.

Others say copper may relieve pain by neutralizing free radicals as the mineral is absorbed through your skin. But you would need to absorb a lot of copper to have that effect, and studies say that's just not possible from a bracelet, especially since many have a lacquer coating that would prevent the copper from reaching your skin.

Arthritis sufferers expect relief

Wearing copper bracelets to calm arthritis symptoms comes from old folk wisdom. Because of the bracelets' popularity, researchers at the Mayo Clinic in Jacksonville, Fla., decided to investigate.

They conducted a randomized, double-blind study involving 610 people with pain in their neck, lower back, elbows, wrists, or feet. For 28 days, half of the study participants wore an ionized bracelet containing 85 percent copper and 15 percent zinc. The other half wore a placebo bracelet.

At the start of the study, 409 participants responded to a survey. When asked whether they believed copper could reduce joint and muscle pain, 80 percent believed it could.

At the end of the study, both groups reported a significant improvement in their pain levels. In fact, there was little difference between the two groups.

Beware of ads that sound too good

Although there is no cure for arthritis, the Arthritis Foundation says consumers spend $2 billion a year for sham arthritis cures, like copper bracelets.

Rheumatologists — doctors who specialize in treating rheumatic diseases, like some types of arthritis — reported that 29 percent of people with pain in the joints, inflammation, stiffness, or muscle soreness had used magnets or copper bracelets. What's more, bracelets came in second to chiropractic care as the most common complementary and alternative medicine used.

---

6 creative ways to cope with RA

Don't become overwhelmed by the pain and exhaustion of rheumatoid arthritis (RA). Add these tips to your arsenal as extra weapons in your fight against arthritis.

- Have faith. A daily spiritual experience puts you in a better mood with less pain.
- Boost your workout. Don't baby your joints after an RA flare. Ask your doctor about cranking up your exercise program.
- Unwind with a massage. It loosens tight muscles and helps you relax. But be careful of inflamed joints since a massage can make them worse.
- Sidestep stiffness. Don't sit in the same position for too long. Get up and move around every so often.
- Plan ahead. Think about the best way to accomplish your daily tasks without stressing your joints.
- Be knowledgeable. Learning about your form of arthritis will give you a better outlook on your future.

If you tend to be susceptible to advertising because you'll do anything to get rid of your pain, ask yourself this question. Would I find out about an incredible medical breakthrough for my arthritis through an ad?

For more information on how to recognize and avoid false and outrageous advertising claims, read *Spot fake cures and false claims* in the introduction, *Crack the code on health claims* on page 2.

Don't wear it — eat it

Copper works as an anti-inflammatory and is an important mineral for arthritis sufferers. Some health professionals recommend getting 2 to 4 milligrams of copper every day to relieve symptoms.

So instead of wearing a copper bracelet, eat foods that are rich in copper, like these:

- Seafood — oysters, lobster, crab, and clams

- Nuts — cashews, macadamia nuts, pecans, almonds, and pistachios

- Legumes — lentils, navy beans, and peanuts

- Chocolate — unsweetened or semisweet baker's chocolate and cocoa

- Black pepper

- Enriched cereals — bran flakes, shredded wheat, and raisin bran

- Fruits and vegetables — dried fruits, mushrooms, tomatoes, sweet potatoes, potatoes, bananas, grapes, and avocados

CoQ10 for Parkinson's

Coenzyme may stave off decline

It sounds more like a "Star Wars" character than a dietary supplement, but CoQ10 may be quite a force when it comes to fighting Parkinson's disease.

This movement disorder affects as many as one million Americans — including celebrities Muhammad Ali and Michael J. Fox. Symptoms include impaired balance and coordination, stiffness, slow movement, and trembling arms, legs, and face.

Parkinson's gets worse with age, but CoQ10 may help slow its progression. Let's see R2D2 or C3PO do that.

How it works

A group of cells in an area of the brain called the *substantia nigra* produce a chemical called dopamine, which is a neurotransmitter or chemical messenger. Dopamine transports signals to the parts of the brain that control movement and coordination.

When Parkinson's disease occurs, these cells begin to malfunction and eventually die, and your brain produces less and less dopamine. That results in a diminishing of motor control in your muscles, which translates into the tremors and instability that mark Parkinson's.

One theory as to why the cells die is that they are damaged by unstable molecules called free radicals. Another theory is that the mitochondria, which are small, energy-producing bodies within the cell, become dysfunctional.

Coenzyme Q-10 (CoQ10) plays an important role in the mitochondria and is also a powerhouse antioxidant. Researchers think it may act in some way on the sick and dying cells that produce dopamine, protecting them from further harm.

More CoQ10 means less disability

The strongest evidence for CoQ10 comes from a recent trial conducted by researchers at the University of California-San Diego.

- Eighty people with Parkinson's disease took either 300 milligrams (mg), 600 mg, or 1,200 mg of CoQ10 per day or a placebo. Everyone in the study also received 1,200 IU per day of vitamin E.

- Researchers used the Unified Parkinson Disease Rating Scale, a common clinical scale, to measure disability throughout the study. People were evaluated for up to 16 months or until they required drug treatment.

Take back your life after Parkinson's

There isn't a cure for Parkinson's disease yet, but you can take steps to help control it naturally.

- Exercise could help delay some of the stiffness and fatigue that Parkinson's can cause. Try aerobics, strengthening exercises, walking, tai chi, or another exercise class.
- Avoid foods that seem to make your symptoms worse, like hot or spicy dishes.
- Limit saturated fat — especially red meat — but get plenty of fiber.
- Ask your doctor if protein-rich foods could interfere with your Parkinson's medication.
- Join a support group for encouragement and helpful advice.
- Consider physical therapy for movement or speech difficulties.
- Eat plenty of foods containing a natural chemical called quercetin. You'll find this brain-saving nutrient in apples, berries, and onions.

- Less disability developed in the people taking CoQ10, with those taking the most reaping the greatest benefit. People taking 1,200 mg of CoQ10 daily lessened the progression of disability by 44 percent compared to those in the placebo group.

While this study fills researchers with hope, they need to confirm these results in a larger study before they can wholeheartedly recommend CoQ10 for Parkinson's disease.

Take wait-and-see approach

You can find CoQ10 in drugstores, health food stores, and supermarkets. It comes in a variety of forms, including soft-gel capsules, tablets, wafers, and hard capsules. Products may contain anywhere from 10 mg to 200 mg per pill.

Only small amounts of CoQ10 are available in foods, so you can't expect to get it from your diet. But you can find some in beef, chicken, mackerel, bran, sesame, beans, spinach, sardines, and peanuts.

Currently, no guidelines exist for CoQ10 intake. But researchers caution against taking the high doses used in the above study until more trials are conducted. Talk with your doctor about supplementing with CoQ10.

Be careful if you take blood thinners or drugs for diabetes. CoQ10 can interact with these drugs. Some medications, like statins, beta blockers, and antidepressants, lower the amount of CoQ10 in your body, so you may need to take more to get any benefit.

The "Co" in CoQ10 could stand for "Costly." Expect to pay $15 to $45 per month for this supplement. Higher doses, such as the 1,200 mg used in the study, can cost as much as $10 a day.

Don't expect any serious side effects, but some people experience heartburn, abdominal pain, nausea, headache, and dizziness.

Until researchers learn more about CoQ10, stick to standard remedies to control Parkinson's symptoms. Common prescription drug treatments include levodopa, levodopa with carbidopa, deprenyl, amantadine, and anticholinergics.

Although it's too early to tell, CoQ10 may prove to be an effective alternative to prescription drugs. Stay on the lookout for the latest research.

Cranberry juice for UTIs

★★★

Red fruit flushes out bacteria

Cranberries — one of only three fruits native to North America — were used by the early American Indians to cure bladder and kidney disorders. The Pilgrims used cranberries in the 17th century to treat a variety of ailments. Prior to antibiotics, the little red berry continued to be a popular remedy for urinary tract infections (UTIs).

Today, cranberries are still a great way to fight urinary tract infections, a condition one in every five American women will suffer at least once in their lives. Eleven million women a year take medicine for UTIs.

How it works

Studies show cranberry juice really can prevent UTIs. It was previously thought the tart little berries work by making your urine more acidic, which slows the growth of bacteria. But today it is generally agreed that cranberries keep infection-causing bacteria from clinging to your urinary tract.

It's been found that compounds in cranberries (and also blueberries) called proanthocyanidins prevent *P-Fimbriated E. coli* bacteria from attaching to the lining. This type of bacterium is a major cause of UTIs. By drinking cranberry juice, you wash away the bacteria before they can start an infection.

Juice prevents resistant bugs, too

Researchers at Rutgers University and the University of Michigan tested this idea of non-stickiness. They found that cranberry juice will not only keep regular bacteria from staying in the urinary tract, it works the same on antibiotic-resistant germs.

The scientists put 39 kinds of UTI-causing *E. coli* into urine collected from women before and after they drank cranberry juice. Then they tested to see if the bacteria would attach to urinary tract cells. Of the 39 different types of germs, 24 were resistant to antibiotics.

Banish bacteria to relieve UTIs

Try these natural remedies to rid your body of infection-causing bacteria.

- Vitamin C-rich fruits and juices make your urine more acidic, and that means bacteria has a harder time growing.
- Water does a great job of washing bacteria out of your system before it has a chance to multiply. If your urine is pale — not dark — you're getting enough.
- Eat parsley for its vitamin C and for the fact it is a diuretic. It will increase urine flow, washing bacteria out of your body.
- Go to the bathroom as soon as you feel the urge. Keeping your bladder empty means there's no place for the bacteria to grow.
- Folklore says to wear cotton panties instead of nylon, and to avoid tight pants and pantyhose. There's no scientific evidence these tips work, but extra precautions can't hurt.
- Avoid douches and bubble baths, and use hypoallergenic pads and tampons — changing them often.

They found that 80 percent of all bacteria and 79 percent of the resistant bacteria would not stick after being in the cranberry urine. All of the bacteria in urine taken before the women drank the juice stuck to the lining of the walls.

Cranberry is prevention, not cure

Plenty of evidence shows cranberries are effective at preventing UTIs. Some studies believe sexually active adult women with recurring UTIs could experience a 50 percent drop in infections by taking either cranberry juice or tablets.

But there is no reliable evidence you can treat infections with cranberry juice. Once the UTI has actually started, you need to see a doctor who can prescribe stronger medicine, like antibiotics. UTIs can become quite serious if they spread to your kidneys.

How much should you take?

Opinions vary on exactly how to get cranberries' good juices into your body. Research has focused on unsweetened cranberry juice, cranberry juice cocktail, and cranberry extract tablets. One recent trial that was positive for UTI prevention used one 300- to 400-milligram tablet twice a day, or 8 ounces of pure unsweetened juice three times a day.

Other dosage recommendations include drinking just 3 ounces of juice per day, but it takes four to eight weeks before benefits take effect. Another suggestion is 8 to 16 ounces per day. The Rutgers-Michigan study — which received funds from Ocean Spray Cranberries, Inc. — gave its subjects 8 ounces of cranberry juice cocktail. It began to work in the urine within two hours and lasted up to 10 hours.

Watch out for special problems

Cranberries seem to be a safe choice for UTI prevention, with only a couple of exceptions.

- It's possible long-term use will increase the risk of oxalate kidney stones for people who have a history of that particular type of stone.

- Doctors in Great Britain think cranberry juice may increase the effect of the blood thinner warfarin, causing internal bleeding and possibly death. Pending further investigation, they say people taking warfarin should stay away from cranberry juice.

Dairy for weight loss

Simple way to burn fat

Americans are 25 pounds heavier than they were in 1960, according to the National Center for Health Statistics — but help may already be in your refrigerator. Raise your metabolism and drop pounds with the calcium in dairy products.

How it works

Scientists suspect calcium helps determine whether you burn fat. When your calcium levels sink too low, your body thinks you're starving, so it stores fat. When calcium is high, you burn fat more efficiently — and perhaps discard more fat in your waste, too. So you might rev up your metabolism and slim down with calcium.

Losing weight may even limit your ability to absorb calcium, according to a recent study of postmenopausal women. And that might mean that older women need extra calcium when they're shedding pounds.

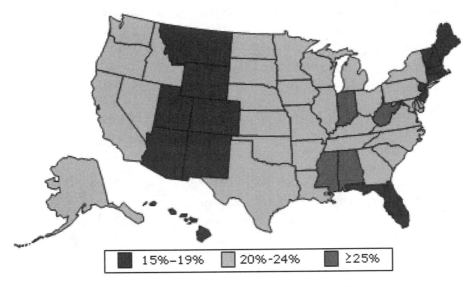

Percentage of state population that is obese.

Watch for more reviews

Two separate reviews examined the research on calcium and weight. Both found enough evidence to conclude that a high calcium intake may help prevent weight gain and may even purge some pounds — but scrimping on calcium might have the opposite effect.

What's more, both reviews agree that dairy calcium seems to have a bigger impact on weight loss than calcium from supplements. Experts think that other dairy ingredients might be pitching in to help.

Yet many clinical human studies have been too small, too short, or funded by the dairy industry. That's why large clinical trials and further research are still needed to help settle issues like how calcium affects weight, how safe and effective it may be, and the best way to use it.

Become a clever calcium consumer

But adding more calcium is probably still a good idea for most of us. After all, more than half of all adults in the U.S. don't get the recommended amount of calcium — which is 1,000 to 1,200 milligrams (mg) per day for older adults. Just adding one to two servings of dairy (from 300 to 600 mg of calcium) to your diet every day, could make a difference in your weight and your health.

While calcium might keep your metabolism from sabotaging your weight, this nutrient isn't a miracle pill. Calcium only helps you lose weight if you're already on a reduced-calorie diet. So add calcium-rich dairy to your meals only if you cut calories somewhere else — and favor dairy choices that are low in fat and calories.

Sure-fire weight loss tips

Weight loss fads come and go. But common sense and a healthy plan of attack will help you melt off the pounds.

- Drink water every day.
- Eat plenty of whole grains, legumes, and fresh fruits and vegetables.
- Cut back on sweets, refined carbohydrates, processed foods, and unhealthy fats.
- Get at least 30 minutes of moderate exercise every day.

If, however, you want some pound-dropping tricks, don't jump on the latest diet craze — try these instead:

- Keep a food diary, writing down everything you eat.
- Sit down to eat, concentrate on your food, and push the plate aside when you're full — whether it's empty or not.
- For a home-grown folk remedy that claims to turn off a craving for sweets, rinse your mouth with a mixture of one teaspoon of baking soda dissolved in a glass of warm water. Be sure not to swallow.

Both dairy lovers and dairy haters can benefit from calcium. If you love dairy, try these easy ways to slip dairy foods into a low-calorie diet.

- Add low-fat milk to your coffee and tea.

- Enjoy a half cup of low-fat frozen yogurt.

- Don't be fooled by sour cream, cream cheese, coffee creamer, or whipped cream. They're all low-calcium wimps.

- Add two servings of low-fat yogurt to your daily menu. Mix in some fruit for a treat.

- Trade in that high-calorie milk shake for a smoothie blended with fruit, ice, and low-fat milk.

- Sprinkle fat-free dry milk powder on almost anything. You won't notice the taste or calories, and 2 tablespoons add about 100 mg of calcium.

If you hate dairy, get calcium from sources like canned sardines with bones, calcium-fortified orange juice, kale, and hearty fortified cereals. While calcium supplements are only about half as effective as dairy products in helping you lose weight, you can also try a daily dose of around 500 mg of calcium citrate.

DASH diet for high blood pressure

★★★

Relief is just a meal plan away

Monitoring your blood pressure is important, especially as you get older. The seventh annual report of the National Committee on Prevention, Detection, Evaluation, and Treatment of High Blood Pressure makes it plain:

- Once you reach 50 years of age and starting with a blood pressure level of 115/75 mmHg, the risk of heart disease doubles with each little increase of 20/10 mmHg.

- Higher than normal blood pressure is the number one attributable risk factor for death around the world.

- Regardless of the medication you take, high blood pressure can only be controlled if you are motivated to stay on your blood-pressure reduction plan.

These are great reasons for giving the DASH diet plan (short for Dietary Approaches to Stop Hypertension) a shot. The fact is, DASH will dramatically lower blood pressure — without additional risky drugs.

It's as simple as these 10 natural steps which involve eating less of some things and more of others:

Fight back with B vitamins

Your heart has a new enemy. Researchers found that an amino acid called homocysteine pairs up with cholesterol to damage your arteries, which can cause a heart attack or stroke.

Luckily, researchers discovered weapons you can use to fight homocysteine. A trio of B vitamins — folic acid, vitamin B6, and vitamin B12 — team up to convert homocysteine into a less-dangerous substance.

Asparagus, beets, spinach, pinto beans, lentils, enriched cereal, and beef liver are good sources of folic acid. Vitamin B12 is found in cottage cheese, sirloin steak, tuna, sardines, and chicken liver. You'll find vitamin B6 in spinach, sweet potato, baked potato, chicken breast, and bananas.

If you drop your B-vitamin defensive line, you can expect a full-scale assault on your arteries. By getting more B vitamins, you'll put heart disease to flight.

- limit salt, trim fat, reduce red meat, settle for fewer sweets and sweet drinks.

- eat more fruit, vegetables, whole grains, lowfat dairy products, poultry, and lean fish.

In short, it's a plan you can live with and enjoy.

How it works

Nutritionist Mary Beth Horrell, with the Diabetes and Health Education Center at Asheville, North Carolina's Mission Hospital, can vouch for the healthfulness of the DASH diet. Her hospital's high blood pressure program has used DASH for years.

When the DASH plan was first investigated, Horrell says, it emphasized limiting fats and sweets and eating well-rounded, nutritious meals. Those who used it saw their blood pressure drop. Then DASH research began to focus on sodium, and blood pressure numbers fell even further. "The final conclusion," says Horrell, "was that both approaches are effective independently, but when combined they have the most beneficial results."

DASH zeroes in on sodium — the main ingredient in salt. "We only need 500 to 1,000 milligrams each day, so most people consume far more than they need," explains Horrell. "It's responsible for maintaining fluid balance. I tell my patients that sodium acts like a sponge and holds on to water. But too much sodium or water in the body causes imbalances.

"Sodium also regulates muscle contractions," she continues, "and, since our heart is a muscle, it can affect how the heart pumps. Our blood pressure is a measure of our heart beating and relaxing."

But reducing sodium isn't merely a matter of throwing the salt shaker away, Horrell says. "DASH is inherently lower in sodium because it emphasizes fresh fruits and vegetables, which have very little sodium."

Horrell believes the DASH plan is here to stay — it works and focuses on moderation. "It doesn't eliminate any food groups. It includes foods that anybody has access to. It's satisfying nutritionally. And people who use it aren't hungry. There aren't any dangers associated with DASH that I'm aware of. DASH makes sense to me."

Studies give DASH the go ahead

Three major studies — DASH, DASH-Sodium, and PREMIER — all support the blood-pressure benefits of the DASH plan. These studies have proven that a diet rich in fruits, vegetables, whole grains, and low-fat dairy products and low in fat, refined carbohydrates, and sodium reduces blood pressure. What's especially exciting is the fact that DASH can lower blood pressure as much as any single blood-pressure medication can — 10, 14, even 16 points or more.

Plan your daily DASH	
Food group	**Daily servings**
grains and grain products	7-8
vegetables	4-5
fruits	4-5
dairy (low-fat or fat free)	2-3
fats and oils	2-3
meats, poultry, and fish	2 or less
nuts, seeds, and dry beans	4-5 per week
sweets	5 per week

These large randomized studies also settled some long-standing debates over whether certain nutrients — like calcium, potassium, and magnesium — were blood-pressure-reducing kingpins. When they were provided in supplement form, they didn't make much difference. But when eaten in the foods of the DASH plan, the blood pressure dropped. In other words, those nutrients work best when they come from natural foods, such as those you eat in the DASH plan.

Help heal your heart with DASH

DASH is more than a diet. It's part of a lifestyle that can better your life. Your health is important, but nobody wants a "grit-your-teeth-I-can't-wait-till-this-is-over" regimen. Coupled with keeping a healthy weight, exercising regularly, and quitting smoking, DASH will help you enjoy a healthy drop in your blood pressure and cholesterol, less fatigue, and a decreased risk of heart disease and osteoporosis.

For a free copy of Facts about the DASH Eating Plan — including a sample week of DASH meals — visit the Web site *http://emall.nhlbihin.net.*

The only warnings you'll need

Beware of sodium. "Sodium hides in everything," warns Horrell. "Salt has about 2,400 milligrams in a single teaspoon. Most processed and canned foods have excessive sodium. When you eat out, it's heavily used — especially in fast foods."

Adjust to more fiber. You may experience some bloating or flatulence if you're not used to eating beans, bananas, and other high-fiber foods at DASH levels, so adjust gradually.

Don't substitute supplements for good food. Get your nutrients from the wholesome, nutrient-rich DASH diet. "Magnesium, calcium, and potassium do lower blood pressure, but this combination taken in supplements doesn't show the same results," Horrell says.

Keep taking your blood-pressure medicine, and don't tamper with your dosage without first consulting your doctor.

And if you slip up and overindulge, don't give up — for your blood pressure's sake.

Bring high blood pressure down naturally

Besides sticking to a healthy eating plan — like the DASH diet — and exercising regularly — like taking daily walks — there are other things you can do to lower your high blood pressure.

- Get enough calcium, magnesium, and potassium — three minerals that really keep your blood pressure in check by balancing nutrients in your body and relaxing your blood vessels.
- Stop smoking. It stiffens your arteries.
- Limit alcohol to no more than two drinks a day for a man, and one drink a day for a woman.
- Increase the amount of omega-3 fatty acids in your body by eating fish and other foods rich in polyunsaturated fats. Your arteries will respond by being much more relaxed and flexible and your heart won't have to work so hard.
- Cook with olive oil for its monounsaturated fat.
- Load up on fiber-rich foods.

DHEA for aging

Hormone falls short of hype

The supplement DHEA has been marketed as the Fountain of Youth in pill form — and millions of Ponce de Leons have spent big bucks on it ever since.

But they're all wet. This popular pill promises a great deal, but has yet to deliver.

How it works

DHEA (dehydroepiandrosterone) is a steroid hormone produced by your adrenal glands. It is sometimes called the "mother" hormone because your body converts it into whatever hormone it needs most at the moment, like testosterone, estrogen, or adrenaline.

Levels of DHEA peak at around age 20 and then decline steadily throughout the rest of your life. In fact, DHEA levels are known to be one of the most reliable measures of aging.

Some scientists think older people may gain back their youthful vitality by increasing the amount of DHEA in their bodies. Because DHEA helps your body produce hormones, it may help improve your mood and memory, boost your sex drive, increase muscle mass, and strengthen your immune system.

Not all of these benefits have been proven, however, and the long-term effects of DHEA supplementation are not known.

Glimmers of hope

Evidence of DHEA's anti-aging benefits remains skimpy, but there have been some positive developments.

- DHEA has shown promise in treating sexual dysfunction in women and impotence in men. There is also preliminary evidence that it helps relieve depression.

- A small Italian study of 20 postmenopausal women showed that 25 milligrams (mg) of DHEA per day might work as well as hormone replacement therapy.

- In a small Japanese study, 24 men received either 25 mg of DHEA or a placebo. Those taking DHEA improved their artery flexibility and insulin sensitivity, which may help protect against heart disease and diabetes.

- DHEA has become an accepted treatment for lupus and other autoimmune disorders.

But these glimmers of hope don't shed enough light on the many questions about DHEA. Right now, experts don't have enough solid evidence to recommend using it.

Consumer help

Doctors may prescribe DHEA for certain conditions, like lupus, but you can also buy it without a prescription. Supplements range from 5 mg to 100 mg per pill.

While people with lupus can safely take up to 200 mg of DHEA per day, the most common daily dose seems to be 25 to 50 mg.

DHEA does not come without risks. Side effects include acne, upset stomach, abdominal pain, high blood pressure, insomnia, hair loss, facial hair growth, voice deepening, and changes in your menstrual pattern.

Slow the wheel of time

Drinking from the Fountain of Youth is really no more mysterious than adapting some good, common-sense approaches to life. If you faithfully follow these nine simple rules, you should look and feel better for many years to come.

- Eat a balanced diet.
- Get 30 minutes of moderate exercise every day.
- Drink lots of water.
- Protect yourself from sun damage.
- Limit alcohol.
- Maintain a healthy weight.
- Get enough deep, restful sleep.
- Take a multivitamin.
- Manage stress.

It may also lower your good HDL cholesterol levels and increase insulin resistance or insulin sensitivity for people with diabetes. Most seriously, DHEA may boost your risk for breast, prostate, or ovarian cancers.

Remember, the long-term safety, effectiveness, and proper dosages of DHEA have not yet been established. Stay away from it unless you have a prescription or your doctor's approval.

Here's a better idea. Face the fact that you're going to get older. Instead of wasting time and money searching for the Fountain of Youth, spend it enjoying life.

Echinacea for colds

Coping with a common virus

Folks have sworn by echinacea's cold-fighting power for generations. Nevertheless, studies are casting doubt on its reputation. Until researchers learn more, there's no harm in giving echinacea a try if you feel a cold coming on.

How it works

When it comes to cold prevention, echinacea has the most established history of all the herbs. Also called the purple coneflower, this member of the daisy family grows in the Midwestern United States. It was used by Native Americans to treat colds, coughs, sore throats, toothaches, and even snakebite.

Scientists thought echinacea could battle colds and flu by boosting your immune system, giving you added ammunition to fight off the attack of a cold virus. Most modern experts agree it may be helpful in treating the early stages of upper respiratory tract infections. However, there is no strong evidence it will help prevent them.

In fact, some recent studies have found that people who took echinacea were no less likely to develop colds than people who took a placebo.

How the herb fared

One study involved students at the University of Wisconsin in Madison. At the first sign of a cold, the 148 volunteers were given either echinacea capsules or a placebo. The students took the capsules for 10 days or until their symptoms disappeared.

A similar study involved 128 people. The participants began taking echinacea within 24 hours of the onset of cold symptoms to see if they recovered faster.

The third was a double-blind, placebo-controlled clinical trial. Its aim was to test the ability of echinacea to prevent a cold. Forty-eight healthy adults received echinacea or a placebo for seven days before and seven days after they were intentionally infected with a virus. Symptoms were monitored to see whether the participants would actually catch a cold after being infected.

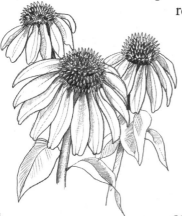

According to these three studies, echinacea had little effect on the cold virus. In the first study, both groups of college students endured their colds an average of six days.

In the second, the time it took for symptoms to disappear among those taking echinacea was not statistically different from those who took the placebo.

New way to fight colds

Colds are easier to catch and harder to shake the older you get. Your immune system just doesn't have the infection-fighting power it had in your younger years. So what can you do to strengthen your defenses and hold off the common cold? Try vitamin E.

A Tufts University study found that taking 200 IU of vitamin E every day improves your chances of avoiding colds. For a year, half of the study participants took vitamin E, while the other half took a placebo.

At the end of the study, the people taking vitamin E had a 20-percent lower risk of catching a cold than those taking the placebo.

In the third study — the one designed to see whether echinacea would prevent people from coming down with a cold — 92 percent of those who took echinacea and 95 percent of those taking the placebo "caught" the virus, but not all of them developed a cold. Fewer people taking echinacea, however, got a cold. Yet, the researchers think this was due to chance.

Not everyone in the medical community thinks these studies paint an accurate picture of echinacea. Some health professionals believe these studies are far from conclusive. They recommend more studies using a larger number of participants with different types of echinacea and dosages.

Use it right if you use it

Herbal experts who promote its use say it's best to combine two types of echinacea — *E. purpurea* and *E. angustifolia*. Look for a brand containing at least 3.5 percent echinacosides, the active ingredient.

At the first sign of a cold, they recommend taking two 100-milligram capsules every four hours, or a teaspoonful of the liquid every two or three hours.

Maintain this dose for the first couple of days, and then cut it in half until your symptoms disappear. Don't use echinacea for longer than eight weeks at a stretch. Also be aware that it can interact with some prescription drugs.

Because of the possibility echinacea might overstimulate the immune system, it could worsen lupus, multiple sclerosis, rheumatoid arthritis, or other autoimmune disorders. Talk with your doctor before using echinacea if you have any of these conditions.

Say goodbye to cold misery

Even when a cold hits you hard, there are plenty of easy, home-grown remedies to help you feel better fast.

- Chicken soup really can break up congestion and boost your immune system.
- Wash your hands. Do it well — with soap and warm water — and do it often.
- Drink, drink, drink. You'll prevent dehydration and thin the mucus in your lungs.
- Whip up a tasty cough syrup by mixing 8 ounces of warm pineapple juice with two teaspoons of honey.
- Get some extra shut-eye. When your body is working to fight off a cold, it needs plenty of rest.
- Drink orange juice, eat strawberries, or take a good multivitamin — but boost your vitamin C and you may reduce the length of time you suffer cold symptoms.
- Gargle with one-half teaspoon of salt stirred into a cup of warm water.

Essential oil therapy for hair loss

Rescue your hair with a massage

God created a few perfect heads — the rest he covered with hair. At least that's what proud bald men like to say. Of course, not everyone agrees with them, especially the many women who experience hair loss.

If you find your head moving a little too rapidly toward "perfection," consider essential oil therapy.

How it works

Essential oils have been used for centuries in a variety of healing ways, such as pain relievers, antiseptics, and sleeping aids. Now they're being considered to help reverse and prevent hair loss. Some researchers theorize the oils might help because of their great ability to penetrate and diffuse into a surface. They believe the oils have the power to vibrate and emit electromagnetic waves.

In a recent study, researchers used essential oils that could stimulate circulation and improve the nutrition intake of the hair cells. The essential oils also regulated the functioning of the oil-secreting glands that contain the hair follicles. Researchers think it's possible the oils helped create better conditions for cell division to take place.

Thin evidence for thicker hair

Few studies have tested essential oil therapy, but the following two trials paint a promising picture.

A French study examined male-pattern baldness, which affects half of all men by age 50 and 25 percent of white women between the ages of 35 to 45. The combination of essential oils and an electromagnetic field three times a week for 26 weeks prevented hair loss and increased hair density. Despite the positive results, this treatment, which involved a special helmet that delivered electromagnetic pulses for half an hour, might not be very practical.

A preliminary study of essential oils alone showed some success in preventing hair loss, but not much in growing new hair.

In Scotland, researchers tested aromatherapy on people with alopecia areata, a condition that causes your hair to fall out in patches. Half of those in the study massaged thyme, rosemary, lavender, and cedarwood essential oils, mixed with "carrier" oils, into their scalps each day. The other half used just the carrier oils — grapeseed and jojoba.

Lock in your locks

Since there are various medical reasons for hair loss, get a checkup to rule all of them out before you go to Plan B.

- Ask your doctor to check your hormones since they can affect how quickly, or thickly, your hair grows.
- Have your blood tested for iron and thyroid levels.
- Discuss all medications with your doctor. Antidepressants, birth control pills, blood thinners, and gout medicine are possible hair loss culprits.
- Talk to him about recent injuries, infection, fevers, surgery, or even emotional stress. They all can cause hair fallout.

A balanced diet promotes healthy hair growth. On the other hand, drastic weight loss or an extremely low-calorie diet can make your hair fall out.

Finally, take care of the hair you've got. Don't overprocess it with chemicals, harsh treatments, and heat. Buy quality, moisturizing products and see a professional hair stylist regularly.

After seven months, 44 percent of those using essential oils showed improvement in hair growth. Only 15 percent of the other group improved. However, the success could just be due to remission, which occurs in half the people who have recently developed alopecia areata.

While the evidence for essential oil therapy remains rather sparse, it might be worth a try. After all, what do you have to lose except more hair?

Whip up your own treatment

Hair today, gone tomorrow? Try this hair root stimulator and get out your comb.

You'll need two drops each of thyme and cedarwood essential oils and three drops each of lavender and rosemary essential oils. As for carrier oils, which dilute the essential oils to prevent irritation, use 3 milliliters (mL) of jojoba oil and 20 mL of grapeseed oil.

Blend the oils together and massage into your scalp for two minutes each night. Wrap your head in a warm towel to help the skin absorb the oils.

It might get expensive to keep up this treatment for a long time, and there's no guarantee of success. However, the massage might make you feel — and smell — good.

Look for essential oils in herb shops, health food stores, and drugstores.

Exercise balls for fitness

★ ★ ☆

Strengthen 'core' muscles

Here's a new way to flatten your stomach without gut-wrenching exercises to turn ugly flab into rock-hard abs. It's a giant inflatable ball called an exercise ball — or a stability, Swiss, physio, or Sissel ball.

The latest rage is to do crunches on an exercise ball. You can now abandon sit-ups for the less demanding but more effective curl-up or crunch. It's an easy exercise to flatten your bulging belly and strengthen your back and stomach muscles.

Physical therapists from Germany and Switzerland have long used the balls for sports training and rehabilitation. And many therapeutic and athletic conditioning professionals have been using these "Swiss balls" since the late 1980s. Today they are a staple for personal trainers and health clubs.

How it works

Crunches aren't the only exercises that can be done with the balls. They are used for everything from push-ups to calf stretches to strength training. Most typically involve sitting or lying on the ball, both face up and face down.

The ball's key advantage for exercise is its instability. The ball requires you to balance yourself while exercising, which forces you to use a variety of muscles, particularly in the "core" area of your abdomen, back, and hips.

So while you're working out your arms or legs, you're also strengthening these important parts of your body. Core conditioning helps prevent back pain and other injuries and allows you to perform everyday activities more easily.

Does it really help?

How much good a stability ball does depends on whom you ask and what you're using it for. Training journals and press releases suggest considerable benefits, but scientific evidence isn't quite as enthusiastic. Studies have shown that:

- Abdominal muscles get a better workout when crunches are done on exercise balls.

- Rugby players who trained with exercise balls suffered fewer low back and groin injuries.

- Swimmers and runners improved their core stability but didn't improve their race times.

The general conclusion is that you're not going to get stronger arms and legs from instability training, but you can get a stronger torso — core stability — and better balance and posture.

Get fit for life

Studies show regular exercise can reverse 20 years of aging. If that doesn't motivate you to start getting fit, nothing will. Here are some important steps on your quest for a healthier you.
- Pick an exercise regimen that fits your budget and lifestyle.
- Consider hiring a trainer for a one-on-one session to make sure you're doing everything right.
- Take a class.
- Start small. Plan three 10-minute sessions throughout the day. Soon, you'll be able to do more.
- Stretch.
- Ideally, your workout will raise your heart rate. Talk to your doctor about what is a safe target heart rate for you.
- Get extra motivation from an exercise group or buddy.
- Stop exercising and consult your doctor if you experience joint pain, extreme fatigue, dizziness, difficulty breathing, nausea, or chest, arm or shoulder pain.

Don't jump on too soon

There is an infinite number of exercises you can do on an exercise ball, but a great many of them are designed for physical therapy rehabilitation or training for athletic events. The difficulty level can be adjusted by changing either the exercise or the air pressure in the ball. It helps to work with an experienced trainer.

Normal fitness benefits from these balls are centered mostly on abdominal training. Not surprisingly, improved muscle tone in your abs helps with everyday tasks and prevents back pain. But it's best to get some experience with the exercise on solid ground before doing it on an exercise ball.

Fiber for weight loss

★ ★ ★

Slim down smoothly with roughage

Chances are you need to add some fiber to your diet. The average American eats only about 17 grams per day. That's around half the recommended amount. But the fact is, fiber is plentiful in healthy fruits, vegetables, and grains, and you can eat as much of it as your body can handle.

When the VA Medical Center in Lexington, Kentucky compared eight diets — including the popular Atkins and Zone diets — they declared low-fat, high-fiber eating plans the healthiest.

The best news — if you're trying to lose weight, fiber-rich foods will soon become your new best friend.

How it works

Fiber is divided into two main types — soluble and insoluble. Soluble fiber dissolves in water and becomes sticky in your digestive system. This characteristic slows down glucose absorption and helps lower cholesterol. Insoluble fiber doesn't digest. It moves quickly through your intestines, helping to keep you regular. Here's the secret to naturally block out calories from foods — just add fiber to your diet and watch the weight melt away.

- When fiber passes through your body without being digested, it provides little to no calories. Choosing fiber-rich foods instead of fats or sweets can make a big difference in your calorie intake.

- According to the USDA, increasing fiber decreases the digestibility of protein and fat so you end up absorbing fewer calories from these sources.

- Fiber also absorbs water and swells, making you feel full. Soluble fiber even slows the movement of food through your upper digestive tract, so you feel full longer. This means you're less likely to snack between meals.

> You can lose weight without even trying. At the University of Kentucky College of Medicine, 24 men ate canned beans — a good source of fiber — for three weeks. Even while consuming the same total number of calories they lost weight. Amazingly, this 50-cent meal lowered their cholesterol, too.

Find weight loss success with fiber

The evidence for fiber as a weight-loss aid is overwhelming. But perhaps one of the largest and longest studies was conducted by Harvard researchers.

They tracked close to 75,000 healthy, middle-aged women for 12 years and found those who ate the most high-fiber, whole-grain foods gained less weight than those who ate the most refined grains. In addition, the women who increased their intake of fiber or whole grains the most, were half as likely to become obese over the 12-year period.

Tips for a high-fiber day

For your body to function at its peak, the American Dietetic Association says people over 50 should get 20 to 30 grams of both kinds of fiber per day. Younger people need 25 to 35 grams. Some experts recommend even more. The bottom line is, you need to set a daily fiber goal. Experts have found people with a target amount in mind are more likely to reach it than those who just vaguely aim to increase their fiber.

But be careful. Adding too much fiber to your diet too quickly can lead to uncomfortable bloating and gas. So start slowly and drink lots of fluids.

The first meal of the day provides plenty of ways to get high-fiber foods, like oatmeal, fruit, or whole-grain cereal, into your diet. In fact, Michigan State researchers found that women who ate cereal had significantly lower Body Mass Indexes (BMI) — perhaps because they ate less fat and more

Fill up without filling out

Trick your body into losing weight. Here's a strategy that melts off fat safely, naturally, and best yet, easily.

Studies show that people tend to eat the same amount of food, regardless of calories. So instead of trying to limit how much you eat, pay attention to your food's energy density. That means the number of calories in each gram.

The more fiber or water in a food, for instance, the lower its energy (or calorie) density. You'll feel more satisfied after eating it — but you'll be getting fewer calories.

For example, soups have a low energy density because of their high water content. Vegetables are less energy dense than, say pasta.

Another trick is to beat foods. Turn ice cream into a milkshake, to add air, and you'll be more satisfied with less.

By choosing low-energy-dense foods, you could lose weight while eating as much — or more — than you do now.

Fiber heroes and fiber zeroes

Cereals — fiber heroes	Grams of fiber per serving
Kellogg's All-bran original	8.8
Wheatena (cooked with water)	6.6
Kellogg's Raisin Bran	7.3
Kellogg's Frosted Mini-Wheats bite-size	5.5
General Mills Raisin Nut Bran	5.1
General Mills Total Raisin Bran	5.0
Cereals — fiber zeroes	**Grams of fiber per serving**
Kellogg's Corn Flakes	0.7
General Mills Rice Chex	0.3
General Mills Honey Nut Chex	0.3
Kellogg's Corn Pops	0.2
Kellogg's Rice Krispies	0.1
General Mills Reese's Puffs	0.0

fiber. So, if you want to lose weight fast, don't forget to eat a healthy breakfast.

Good sources of fiber include fruits and vegetables — especially with their skin, whole grains, beans, peas, seeds, wheat bran, oat bran, oats, barley, rye, and brown rice.

You can also take fiber supplements, like Metamucil, for an added boost.

Flaxseed for high cholesterol

★★☆

Guard your arteries with a seed

Don't wait until your doctor tells you your arteries are clogged. Start controlling your cholesterol now. Discover how flaxseed can help you take the first step.

How it works

Your liver makes the cholesterol your body needs, but extra cholesterol from the food you eat can lead to dangerous artery-clogging plaque — and maybe a heart attack.

What you need is a secret weapon to snatch extra cholesterol away from arteries before more plaque develops — a sort of natural Roto-rooter that can help keep your arteries cleaned out.

Consider a 10,000-year-old remedy. Scientists aren't really sure how it works, but they think three components in flaxseed might help.

"I personally think fiber is the most important component based on my own research today," says Dr. Philippe Szapary, assistant professor of medicine at the University of Pennsylvania School of Medicine.

Fiber, in grains like flaxseed, helps cut damaging LDL (low-density lipoprotein) cholesterol. That's because fiber nabs bile acids. These bile acids, necessary for digestion, are made from cholesterol. And, like a good security guard, fiber escorts those bile acids right out of your body.

So the next time your body needs to make more bile acids, it pulls cholesterol out of your blood. Less cholesterol in your blood means lower cholesterol readings.

Flaxseed also contains special plant chemicals called lignans. In fact, flaxseed is the richest source of the lignan secoisolariciresinol diglucoside or SDG. Your stomach breaks down SDG into two substances called enterodiol and enterolactone. Because these seem to help lower cholesterol in animals, scientists suspect they might do the same for people.

"The other component is ALA — alpha-linolenic acid," says Szapary. "This is a plant-based omega-3 fatty acid that probably doesn't lower cholesterol." But ALA may still help thwart other causes of heart trouble, like blood clots and irregular heartbeats.

> Several studies suggest that high ALA intake might boost prostate cancer risk. More research is needed to determine whether men should avoid foods containing ALA.

Attacks LDL cholesterol

According to one study, cholesterol levels dropped significantly when folks with high cholesterol ate six slices of flaxseed bread a day.

And when Szapary and a colleague reviewed studies on flaxseed and heart disease, they found more evidence that flaxseed could help reduce harmful cholesterol. It's important to note the researchers used one to five tablespoons (15 to 50 grams) a day in their studies to help participants lower their cholesterol.

"Flaxseed oil doesn't have any of the fiber and none of the lignans so you're really only getting the omega-3," says Szapary. "The flaxseed capsules won't have any effect on your cholesterol."

Szapary suggests that adding flaxseed to a diet low in cholesterol and saturated fat could help reduce LDL cholesterol by 5 to 10 percent. That may sound small, but consider this. "If we, as a people in the United States, were all able to lower our LDL cholesterol by 5 percent, we could cut the rate of heart disease and stroke by the same amount," Szapary says.

Get the dirt on flaxseed

So, at last, you have a way to lower your cholesterol levels and keep them down for good. Just remember — if you have any

Grams of alpha-linolenic acid (ALA) per 100 grams (1/2 cup or 3 1/2 ounces) of food			
Food	ALA	Food	ALA
Flaxseed oil	55.0	Spinach, raw	0.9
Flaxseed	17.0	Cod liver oil	0.7
Canola (rapeseed) oil	11.2	Wheat germ	0.7
Walnut oil	10.4	Olive oil	0.7
Soybean oil	7.0	Peanuts	0.6
Wheat germ oil	6.9	Cream, whipping	0.5
Mayonnaise, soybean	4.2	Cheese, cheddar	0.4
Salad dressing, commercial, Italian	3.3	Purslane	0.4
Walnuts, black	3.3	Navy beans, dry	0.3
Sole, lemon	2.0	Pinto beans, cooked	0.3
Margarine, hard, soybean	1.5	Carp	0.3
Oat germ	1.4	Scallop, sea	0.3
Butter	1.2	Barley, bran	0.3
Peanut oil	1.1	Chicken, light meat	trace
Safflower oil	1.0	Shrimp	trace

Tasty little seed fights cancer, too

Researchers are recognizing flaxseed to be a tiny double power-house in disease prevention.

A small University of Minnesota study showed that eating flaxseed might decrease a kind of estrogen associated with breast cancer. What's more, the fiber in flaxseed can help you sweep cancer-causing substances out of your intestines so you're less likely to get colon cancer.

---

health problems, talk with your doctor before using flaxseed. And for best results, read these pointers before you start.

- You can buy flaxseed in health food stores and some grocery stores. Grind the seeds with a coffee grinder and use them immediately.

- Flaxseed is an intense source of fiber. One tablespoon can contain up to 2.2 grams. To avoid gas and indigestion, start small and add flaxseed to your diet gradually.

- Flaxseed contains phytoestrogens, like lignans, which may have estrogen-like effects. The long-term safety of these has yet to be determined.

Flu shots for flu

★★★

Why you need to get one

The flu vaccine would be well worth the annual shot in the arm even if it only prevented the flu. But it does more. This year's vaccine might help you live to see the arrival of next year's flu season.

How it works

A flu shot is the most effective way to prevent influenza or the flu. It packs a dose of an inactivated vaccine containing killed viruses. Your body, in response to the vaccine, produces antibodies that fend off the flu virus. These viruses change from year to year. That's why you should get a flu shot every year.

> The best time to get your annual flu shot is from October through November.

Can you still catch the flu once you've been immunized? It's possible — according to scientists at the Centers for Disease Control and Prevention (CDC). It takes about two weeks for your body to create immunity. It's also possible the flu virus strain in the shot won't match the strain that pays you a visit.

Even so, once you've had the shot, you're pretty safe. Your guard is up. Most important, the flu shot is approved for almost everyone, including people with chronic health conditions.

Studies span the globe

A team of researchers at Veterans Affairs Medical Center in Minneapolis conducted a study involving over 140,000 people age 65 and older. And they kept up with these folks through two flu seasons to see how the flu shot influenced their overall health. These are the results:

- Chances of being hospitalized for flu or pneumonia dropped by 29 to 32 percent.

- Chances of being hospitalized for heart disease fell by 19 percent.

- The overall risk of dying of any cause plummeted by 48 to 50 percent.

These results are consistent with a study at a university hospital in Thailand. This randomized controlled study involved 125 participants with chronic obstructive pulmonary disease (COPD), which includes chronic bronchitis, emphysema, and asthma.

In this study, 62 participants got the flu vaccine, while 63 received a placebo. Researchers found a 30-percent reduction in hospitalizations for all of the respiratory conditions.

The researchers concluded that the flu shots were highly effective at preventing flu-related complications in people with COPD — like difficulty breathing, sore throat, nasal discharge, fever, wheezing, and coughing.

These added benefits are important because the virus doesn't directly cause most flu deaths. Flu victims die from pneumonia, bacterial infections, and other health problems that stem from the virus.

Prime flu-shot candidates

Who needs an annual flu shot? The CDC recommends them for the following people:

- adults age 65 and older and children ages 6 to 23 months
- people between the ages of 2 and 64 who have chronic health conditions
- women who will be pregnant during flu season
- residents of nursing homes and other long-term care facilities
- health care workers directly involved in patient care
- day care workers in contact with children younger than 6 months of age

Don't get a flu shot if you're allergic to hens' eggs or if you're running a fever.

Now, about the rumor you'll get the flu from a flu shot. You won't. The viruses are dead. They can't spread or reproduce. You may feel some soreness at the vaccination site, but that's true for any injection. If you experience mild flu-like symptoms for several days after your flu shot, don't be alarmed. Remember, it's not the flu. Those symptoms will quickly pass.

Pull through when you've got the flu

All you want is relief from the headache, chills, cough, sore throat, stuffy nose, fever, and muscle aches. Here are some natural ways to feel better.

- Get plenty of liquids.
- Take any over-the-counter products that will treat your symptoms and make you feel more comfortable.
- Consider ginseng supplements to boost your immune system. Some experts suggest 100 milligrams twice a day for several months.
- Rest.
- Run a humidifier or sit in a steamy shower to break up your congestion.
- Drink ginger tea to reduce mucus and soothe a sore throat. Place three or four slices of fresh ginger root in a pint of hot water. Simmer for 10 to 30 minutes.
- Try to eat to keep your strength up.
- Cool down a temperature with elderberry extract. It will reduce congestion and help you sweat your fever away.

Garlic for colds

☆ ☆ ☆

Stop sniffles with an herb

Americans suffer as many as 1 billion colds a year, according to some estimates. While cold medicines may mask the symptoms, they're just temporary fixes and can make you drowsy. Your best bet is to avoid the common cold altogether — and some people think garlic can help.

How it works

Garlic's complex chemistry has long been the subject of scientific study. In the last 50 years, researchers have published more than 2,000 scientific papers documenting the herb's potency against bacteria and its possible benefit against many diseases.

Of garlic's more than 100 chemical parts, one of the strongest is allicin, a compound that's released when a clove is crushed. Allicin is what gives off the pungent aroma particular to garlic, as well as its cousins leeks, chives, and shallots.

Research has found it to be a powerful antibacterial and antiviral agent. Evidence shows that allicin and its subcomponent ajoene are the main powerhouses in garlic that fight off cold viruses.

Press for more proof

British researchers put garlic to the test during the height of cold and flu season. They asked 146 volunteers to take one allicin-containing garlic supplement every day for 12 weeks.

During World War II, the Soviet Army used so much garlic as a remedy the herb earned the nickname "Russian penicillin" for its ability to help the body fight off infections, particularly respiratory and digestive infections.

At the end of the study, the people who took a placebo reported 65 colds, but the group that took the garlic supplements only got 24. On top of that, the supplement takers didn't stay sick as long as those in the placebo group.

It's important to note, however, that more than 200 different kinds of viruses can cause the common cold. Participants in the British study surely didn't encounter all of them, so one study isn't enough to make any recommendations. Keep an eye out for the latest research.

Try a clove encounter of the herb kind

Studies by consumer organizations suggest that the amount of allicin you get from garlic supplements varies wildly depending on which brand you try. Some may not supply enough allicin to do you any good. Preparing dishes with fresh garlic is a delicious way to get allicin — without the trouble of swallowing pills.

Experts aren't sure how much you need, but you may be able to eat as many as three cloves a day without experiencing side effects. Just remember — too much garlic can cause heartburn, gas, wheezing, coughing, vomiting, diarrhea, and skin rashes. Cut back on garlic if any of these occur.

> When shopping for garlic, choose firm bulbs with white, papery skin and big, plump cloves. Avoid brown cloves.

Do not store garlic in plastic bags, sealed containers, or direct sunlight. If you keep garlic in a cool, dry place without too much humidity, it can last four to six months. But don't store it in the refrigerator and never freeze it — it turns mushy.

Mince or crush garlic to make the most of its healing powers. Some evidence suggests that waiting 10 minutes between chopping and cooking preserves garlic's active ingredients better than if you cook it right away. Drying and cooking destroys some of garlic's beneficial compounds. Cook the garlic lightly, if at all.

Although garlic is considered a safe herb, some people are allergic. And here's another thing to keep in mind — if you're taking any medication, check with your doctor. Garlic may boost the effects of anticoagulants and dilute the potency of other drugs.

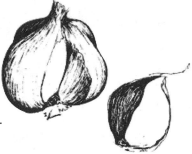

Also ask your doctor about taking garlic supplements or eating garlic if you're scheduled for surgery. Large amounts of garlic could increase bleeding during surgery, so you may need to avoid garlic for a little while.

Garlic for heart disease

Help for your arteries

Garlic might make you wrinkle your nose but that strong smell could keep you healthy. Allicin, the substance that makes the distinctive garlic odor, might help protect your heart and arteries.

How it works

Allicin, a compound that's released when a clove of garlic is crushed, might help reduce high cholesterol. Scientists suspect it shuts down some of the ingredients your body needs to make cholesterol.

Allicin may also lower high blood pressure. By slashing cholesterol and preventing clogged arteries, your blood can zip through with less "oomph" from your heart. Another garlic substance, ajoene, may help thin the blood and prevent clots that could threaten your heart.

The verdict is still out

While at least 10 studies have found that garlic may help foil platelet clumping, an early stage of blood clots, many short-term studies have suggested that garlic has little or no effect on cholesterol levels. Studies on blood pressure seem to find little or no effect, as well.

Yet, many researchers aren't ready to throw in the towel. They say because of the way many of the studies were designed, no firm conclusions can be drawn. More accurate research is needed.

One problem could be allicin. This compound breaks down in the bloodstream so quickly scientists can't measure the amount of allicin in the blood. And, according to a test tube study on garlic supplements used in clinical trials, researchers found only 2 to 18 percent of the allicin promised on the supplements' labels. This could mean garlic study participants got much less allicin than researchers thought.

Fresh garlic doesn't have allicin. But when you chop or crush it, garlic's alliinase enzyme and alliin make allicin. "If you ever baked a big bulb and you can just smear it on like butter and the bite is gone — well that's basically because you couldn't make the allicin any more," says Gardner. High heat cooking is to blame.

Many garlic studies had other flaws. For example, some high cholesterol studies examined people who didn't have high cholesterol. Similarly, research on high blood pressure often studied people with normal blood pressure.

To overcome research problems like these, Christopher Gardner, Ph.D., of Stanford University's Prevention Research Center is conducting a clinical trial. The six-month study is measuring the

> ## Eat food that won't break your heart
>
> "The only time I really got garlic — when I grew up in New Hampshire — was on white bread with butter. That was our garlic bread," says Christopher Gardner, Ph.D., of the Stanford Prevention Research Center. "I bet the butter and the white bread wiped out anything the garlic was doing for me."
>
> Don't erase garlic's benefits by getting too much saturated fat and salt — especially when eating Italian food. Trade cream- and cheese-based sauces, like Alfredo and carbonara, for marinara, wine, or clam sauces. Switch from lasagna or cheese-stuffed pastas to pasta primavera. And don't be fooled by Parmesan cheese or eggplant parmigiana. They can sneak in plenty of saturated fat.

cholesterol-lowering effects of two types of garlic supplements and fresh garlic in food.

Both supplements and food have undergone periodic tests to confirm allicin content, and all 220 study participants have high cholesterol. Stay tuned for the results of this important study.

Try a Chinese approach

"I would really bet garlic has a modest benefit," Gardner says. And perhaps it's one of those 20 or 30 or 50 things that have health benefits. And if you put all those things together, perhaps they add up to an even bigger impact, he suggests.

"Traditional Chinese medicine has used garlic for thousands of years," says Gardner. "They didn't use garlic pills. They used real garlic."

That may be your best bet, too. The clinical trials that tested fresh garlic for atherosclerosis or high cholesterol used 2 to 4 grams of fresh garlic a day — about one clove.

So add garlic to an Asian vegetable stir-fry, a Mediterranean salad, or another heart-healthy dish. If Gardner is right, you might reap extra rewards.

But talk with your doctor first if you take medication. Some drugs, like blood thinners, can be affected by garlic. If your doctor gives you a green light for garlic, don't overdo it. Too much garlic can cause side effects, including heartburn, gas, wheezing, coughing, vomiting, diarrhea, and skin rashes. If you notice any of these, cut back on the garlic.

Thinking of buying garlic supplements? Recently, a consumer organization tested the quality of supplements. They found that the amount of allicin you get from the recommended daily serving of each brand varied wildly.

Ginkgo for leg cramps

★★☆

Banish aches with ancient herb

Muscle cramps can put a kink in your routine, but that's not all. Leg pain that strikes while you walk could be a sign of intermittent claudication (IC), the second stage of peripheral arterial occlusive disease (PAOD).

You don't have to take the pain lying down. An ancient remedy could help you stand up and fight back.

How it works

Doctors usually prescribe daily exercise for intermittent claudication. But it's hard to work out when you can barely walk, and many people with IC give up.

That's where ginkgo biloba comes in. PAOD results from poor circulation in your legs due to clogged arteries. At first, you may feel cramps in your calves, thighs, or buttocks while walking that go away when you sit down. As PAOD progresses, your muscles will cramp at rest, too. Without treatment, you can develop sores on your legs and even gangrene.

"The problem is considerable and growing," says Dr. John Farquhar, professor of Medicine and Health Research and Policy at Stanford University's School of Medicine. Christopher Gardner, his colleague and an assistant professor at Stanford's University's School of Medicine, agrees. "Finding some treatment of benefit is of great importance to the millions who have, or will soon develop, this disorder."

Ginkgo improves your circulation, and it may help you walk farther before the pain strikes, which in turn speeds your recovery from PAOD.

The two experts believe the primary action of ginkgo is to open up, or dilate, some of the smaller arteries in the legs. Cholesterol gradually builds up inside your arteries, making them harder and narrower. That means less blood can squeeze through.

You may not notice the difference until you move. Working muscles need more oxygen and nutrients than resting ones. But if your arteries are blocked, not enough blood can flow through to feed them. The result — your leg muscles starve and begin to cramp up.

Ginkgo may help widen your arteries. Endothelial cells lining the walls of healthy arteries secrete nitric oxide, a chemical that widens and relaxes the blood vessels. Farquhar and Gardner believe this herb somehow increases the amount of nitric oxide in your arteries.

Ginkgo is a powerful antioxidant, so it may neutralize dangerous free radicals before they attack this helpful chemical. Or it may simply increase the amount of nitric oxide your blood vessels produce. Either way, you end up with wider arteries, better circulation, and — hopefully — fewer leg cramps.

Get moving again with ginkgo

Mounting evidence suggests this herbal remedy could be a valuable treatment for IC. In 2004, scientists reviewed nine, strong clinical trials on ginkgo for intermittent claudication. Each trial:

- was double-blinded and randomized.

- tested ginkgo against a placebo.

- used EGb 761, one of the highest-quality ginkgo supplements available.

All nine studies found the herbal extract more effective than placebo for intermittent claudication. What's more, other studies show the herb is just as effective as pentoxifylline, the drug

---

Shape up to shake IC

Herbs may offer hope, but lifestyle changes — not little magic pills — are still the surest way to bounce back from intermittent claudication (IC).

- Stop smoking. The progression of peripheral arterial occlusive disease (PAOD), the condition that causes IC, is directly related to how much you smoke. Quit, and you will improve both your prognosis and how far you can walk pain-free.
- Exercise daily. The best therapy for IC is exercise. Take it in small steps. Walk until you feel pain. Stop, rest until it goes away, then start walking again. Over time, you will be able to walk farther with fewer cramps.
- Control other conditions. Get a grip on high cholesterol, high blood pressure, and diabetes. These can lead to IC and make it worse.

---

doctors often prescribe for IC. Some experts say it's also safer and has fewer side effects.

Gardner, Farquhar, and a team of researchers at Stanford University are currently conducting a rigorous clinical trial on ginkgo biloba for intermittent claudication. They are hopeful but cautious. "The outlook is promising. We now recommend ginkgo for intermittent claudication, but we will wait until our study is complete before we do so with enthusiasm."

Recipe for success

These two experts offer their own prescription for using ginkgo for IC.

- Take 60 milligrams (mg) of ginkgo extract three times a day for intermittent claudication. It may take four to six months to see an improvement.

- If it helps, stay on it for at least a few years. During that time, your body may build new blood vessels in your legs, increasing circulation.

- If your body forms new blood vessels, it might be possible to taper your ginkgo dose, and maybe even stop using it after a few years.

- Look for the brand Ginkgold made by Nature's Way. At the moment, this is the only one Farquhar and Gardner recommend because they don't believe any other brand can make the claim to be EGb 761, the extract used in most clinical trials.

> A small German study suggests a higher dosage may help even more. After six months of treatment, researchers found that people who took a total of 240 mg of ginkgo a day could walk nearly twice as far without pain as those getting 120 mg of the herb daily.

Ginkgo is considered a safe supplement with few side effects. Still, you need to heed a few precautions.

- The herb thins your blood, so avoid it if you are already on blood-thinning medications, such as aspirin or warfarin.

- Stop taking it at least 36 hours before undergoing surgery.

- Use it only under your doctor's supervision. She can help you watch for side effects and decide when to increase or decrease your dosage.

Finally, don't expect this herb to cure you. It may improve IC symptoms, but exercise is key to a full recovery. "Ginkgo is best used as a co-therapy with exercise since exercise is currently the best treatment available," Farquhar and Gardner explain. "Exercise should never be abandoned."

And talk with your doctor about long-term dietary changes to keep your heart and arteries healthy.

Ginkgo for memory loss

Brain booster still unproven

Ginkgo biloba, touted as first aid for a failing memory, is one of the hottest herbs on the market. While scientific theory supports these claims, the evidence does not — yet.

This supplement shows promise for perking up your recall, but it may not work for everyone, or for all forms of memory loss.

How it works

Ginkgo dilates, or widens, blood vessels throughout your body and keeps the platelets in your blood from clumping together. These actions increase your circulation, shipping more oxygen and nutrients to hungry brain cells, or neurons. In theory, this helps them perform at their peek.

It may also protect them. Over time, unstable molecules known as free radicals can damage many of your healthy cells, including neurons. Ginkgo contains free radical fighters called antioxidants — power-packed molecules that disarm free radicals, rendering them stable and harmless before they ravage cells.

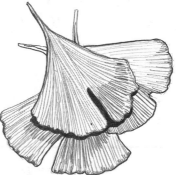

Some experts suspect ginkgo biloba's combination of antioxidant protection and increased circulation could improve both your memory and attention span. But as with many herbal remedies, science has yet to prove it works beyond a shadow of a doubt.

Hope for tomorrow

German researchers reviewed eight good clinical trials on gingko for memory loss. All the trials used LI 1370, a high-quality ginkgo extract. People took either an average of 150 milligrams (mg) of the herb or a placebo each day for six to 12 weeks. Seven of the eight studies showed the herb enhanced people's memory and concentration more than the placebo.

This sounds like solid evidence, but these studies lumped together people with true dementia and those with occasional forgetfulness.

Experts say ginkgo biloba might help dementia, which would explain some positive results, but it may do nothing for passing forgetfulness.

What's more, a new clinical trial found the herb did not boost memory any more than a placebo in healthy seniors without dementia — nor does it seem to treat Alzheimer's disease.

Still, some scientists are hopeful. Most trials have tested this herb in people who already suffer memory loss. But researchers working on a large, well-designed trial funded by the National Institutes of Health hope to discover if it can actually prevent memory loss. Their findings may make or break the case for ginkgo.

Think safety first

One of those researchers, Dr. John Robbins, a professor of medicine at the University of California, Davis, does not yet

---

Stay razor-sharp with good diet

You'll find it's easier to maintain a keen memory if you make smarter food choices.

- Experts say low levels of B vitamins can mean poor memory and problem-solving skills.
  So, eat spinach, beets, avocados, asparagus, low-fat cheese, fish, poultry, potatoes, and beans and you'll get plenty of folate, B12, B6, and thiamin.
- Don't let an iron deficiency impair your mind. Fabulous iron-rich foods like meat, legumes, and green leafy vegetables will help you concentrate and keep you sharp.
- Studies conducted at Massachusetts Institute of Technology showed just one cup of coffee improved mental functioning, reaction time, concentration, and accuracy.
  Drink one cup in the morning for greatest mental alertness. The effects will last for several hours, so you don't need to drink coffee continuously throughout the day. However, you may want to have another cup in the afternoon to combat that after-lunch slump.

---

recommend ginkgo for plugging holes in a leaky memory. "I doubt it will do any harm, except to your bill fold," he notes, "but be careful you get it from a reputable source. What is sold as ginkgo is not regulated in the United States."

So far, Robbins says, no one in his study has suffered major side effects. However, he warns you should check the label of whatever supplement you choose. "Some products sold as ginkgo leaf may contain seeds or bark, which might be harmful." Make sure yours is made solely from the leaves of the tree, the part that packs the medicinal punch. You can find more advice on picking a ginkgo product in *Ginkgo for tinnitus* (see below) and *Ginkgo for leg cramps* on page 158.

Talk with your doctor before using ginkgo for forgetfulness. She can test you for serious conditions, like Alzheimer's, and help you watch for supplement side effects. Be aware it could trigger bleeding if you take it alongside aspirin, heparin, warfarin, or other blood-thinning medications.

Ginkgo for tinnitus

Take a break from constant noise

Ringing, buzzing, hissing, chirping — the noise in your head can drive you to distraction, especially if you suffer from tinnitus. Experts have long said there's no cure, but an herbal remedy may offer resounding relief — if you know how to use it.

How it works

Tinnitus isn't a disease. It's a collection of symptoms with several possible causes, including reduced blood flow in your inner ear.

Your inner ear contains tiny cells shaped like hairs that turn sound vibrations into electrical impulses. The pulses travel to your brain, which interprets them as sounds.

Ginkgo isn't the only answer to tinnitus problems. Talking with a counselor and others who have it can also help. Organizations like the American Tinnitus Association (ATA) offer support groups, information about the condition, and advice on coping with it. Visit them online at *www.ata.org* or call toll-free 1-800-634-8978.

These hair cells need a nutrient-rich supply of blood to stay healthy. Too little blood moving through your inner ear means the cells become sick and die.

Damaged hair cells simply don't work as well as healthy ones. They short-circuit and begin sending constant, nonsense signals to your brain, even when there is no sound. "Your brain picks that up as a ring. That's how we hear it," explains Dr. Michael Seidman, director of the Otologic/ Neurotologic Surgery Division and medical director for the Center for Integrative Medicine at Henry Ford Health System.

Increasing the blood flow in your inner ear may heal these hairs, says Seidman. "If you can improve the blood supply, then perhaps you can improve the tinnitus." Enter ginkgo. It improves your circulation by dilating, or widening, blood vessels and keeping platelets from forming clots.

Mixed results leave questions

In early studies, the herb showed promise as a tinnitus treatment, but its stardom started to wane as larger, more thorough clinical trials ensued.

- A small study in the 1980s showed ginkgo extract completely cured tinnitus symptoms in 35 percent of people tested.

- Not so, says a newer, larger British trial. Out of 720 people, half took 150 milligrams (mg) of ginkgo each day for 12 weeks, and half took a placebo pill. The herb faired no better than placebo.

- A new meta-analysis compiled the results of five placebo-controlled, double-blind trials of the herb for tinnitus. Overall, ginkgo seemed to work no better than placebo.

- But another recent review found ginkgo did indeed improve tinnitus symptoms more than placebo in eight controlled clinical trials.

Why the discrepancies? Seidman says some studies use too low a dosage to have any effect. The British study's 150 mg a day is less than a third of what he prescribes. In addition, tinnitus can have many underlying causes. Ginkgo does not treat all of them, so it won't work for everyone.

Clever ways to silence symptoms

Head noise just annoys some people. For others, it destroys their lives. Before tinnitus drives you crazy, seek help from your doctor and try this advice.

- Just relax. Stress worsens tinnitus, which in turn makes you more anxious. Break the cycle. Yoga, meditation, and visualization are proven ways to manage stress. And anxiety medications such as alprazolam may actually relieve tinnitus symptoms.
- Avoid total quiet. Background noise from a fan, TV, or radio static may cover up tinnitus enough for you to live with it. Turn your kitchen faucet on full blast and listen. If your symptoms seem quieter, then masking may work for you.
- Get a hearing aid. Sometimes the ringing seems loud because you have trouble hearing outside sounds. In fact, tinnitus often accompanies hearing loss. A hearing aid may help you tune into the noise around you and tune out the sounds in your head.

As an authority on tinnitus, Seidman has seen a wide range of response to ginkgo. "If used in the dosage I recommend, probably 10 percent of my patients are nearly cured." Another 10 percent may see no effect, he says, while the other 80 percent experience some, but not total, relief.

Supplement know-how

Even skeptical experts say the herb could be worth a shot, especially if nothing else has helped. "There are no cures for tinnitus, we know that," Seidman says. "But many things may help some patients."

Ginkgo could be one of them. Ask yourself these questions to decide if this herb could help you.

- Does tinnitus interfere with your sleep?
- Does it affect your day-to-day activities?
- How bad are your symptoms on a scale of one to 10, with 10 being the worst?

If you answered "no" or "not much" to the first two questions, and if you rated your symptoms a six or below, you probably have moderate tinnitus, which might benefit from ginkgo. People with more severe tinnitus should seek help from an expert, such as an otolaryngologist — an ear, nose, and throat doctor.

Seidman prescribes 240 mg of ginkgo twice a day for four months to his tinnitus patients. "If it hasn't been effective after four months, it's probably not going to be," he says.

If your tinnitus does improve, he suggests gradually lowering your dosage to find out exactly how much you need. When your ringing returns, increase your dosage again just enough to treat your symptoms.

The supplement you buy can make a difference. Seidman prefers Arches Tinnitus Relief Formula. You can buy others, but check the label for a few key ingredients.

- Look for the words "50 to 1 concentrate" and "tannin-free."

- Make sure it's made from the leaves of the tree and not the bark or seeds, which can be harmful.

- Buy a supplement with at least 24-percent ginkgo flavonoid glycosides and 6 percent terpene lactones.

He also suggests shopping at small health food stores. "They often know what they're doing. I get nervous buying supplements from a drugstore."

Take care — combining ginkgo with other blood-thinning drugs, such as heparin or warfarin, could lead to excessive bleeding. Tell your doctors you take this herb so they avoid prescribing medicines that interact with it.

Ginseng for high cholesterol

Antioxidant help for your arteries

Ginseng has been a busy little herb for the last few thousand years. Its Latin name, *Panax ginseng*, comes partly from panacea, a Greek word that means all-healing. And it's easy to see how ginseng got that name.

How it works

This popular Oriental herb is used throughout America for lowering cholesterol with the added benefits of a stronger immune system and more energy.

Ginseng may lessen stress, relieve fatigue, and improve your memory and concentration. It can also increase your strength and stamina and regulate your blood sugar.

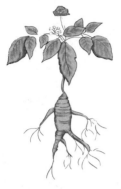

Best of all, ginseng may protect your heart and blood vessels. It unleashes antioxidants, which can fight free radicals that damage your arteries. Ginseng also jumps in to prevent platelets from ganging up into clots that can cause heart attacks.

And perhaps you need worry no more about high cholesterol with this powerful little root. Some herbal experts think ginsenosides, ginseng root's most active ingredients, help your liver snatch up cholesterol particles before they can wreak havoc in your bloodstream.

What's more, ginseng contains a substance called sitosterol. Your intestines absorb sitosterol, which could help slash cholesterol, too.

Research looks encouraging

Even though past studies and reports suggest that ginseng helps control cholesterol, results from animal research have been mixed.

But recently, a study found that eight male college students lowered total cholesterol, harmful LDL cholesterol, and triglycerides after taking ginseng extract for just eight weeks. In addition, their levels of heart-helping HDL cholesterol rose.

This study was brief and had few participants, but it's an encouraging start. More research is needed to verify the study's results, to find out whether ginseng can work safely for everyone, and to see how long it might control cholesterol.

Learn the facts before you buy

If you decide to take ginseng supplements, check with your doctor first. Ginseng isn't for everyone. Although it could help cut your cholesterol, if you have high blood pressure or low blood sugar, this herb might make your problems worse. Ginseng can drive blood pressure up or blood sugar down. It can also make trouble by teaming up with insulin or drugs that reduce blood sugar.

Other side effects include nausea, diarrhea, insomnia, headaches, or low blood pressure.

Don't use ginseng if you are taking warfarin (Coumadin), phenelzine (Nardil), or nifedipine. Also, don't take ginseng with large amounts of caffeine or other stimulants.

Before you buy ginseng supplements, read the label carefully. *Panax ginseng* — also called Asian ginseng — is one of the "true" ginsengs, not an imitator often passed off for the real thing, and it's the most well-researched.

Recently, a major consumer organization tested 18 brands of ginseng supplements. Only one harbored contaminants, but another failed to match the potency claimed on its label. To avoid these problems, look for ginseng supplements that feature the Consumer Labs Seal of Approved Quality on the container.

> You'll find more than one kind of ginseng at the store, so choose wisely. If the bottle promises you *Panax ginseng* or Asian ginseng, you're on the right track. American ginseng or *Panax quinquefolius L.* is generally considered milder than Asian ginseng.

Also, look for an extract labeled "standardized" that contains at least 3 percent total ginsenosides — or 30 milligrams (mg) per gram. Herbal experts recommend taking 100 mg once or twice daily. If you stick with standardized *Panax ginseng* extract, the twice daily dose should provide at least 6 mg of ginsenosides.

Glucosamine for osteoarthritis

⭐ ⭐ ⭐

Rebuild rusty joints

Pop a pain reliever when your arthritic joints act up and you may feel better, but you won't be doing anything to stop the crippling affects of osteoarthritis (OA). Make glucosamine supplements part of your daily routine, however, and you can rebuild your damaged cartilage and strengthen your body's repair system.

> Don't measure how well glucosamine is working by the amount of pain relief you notice. Long-term studies show glucosamine slows cartilage loss, regardless of any change in symptoms.

How it works

Glucosamine occurs naturally in your body and is a major building block of cartilage, the rubbery tissue on the ends of your bones.

When you suffer from osteoarthritis, you experience major chemical changes and physical breakdowns. For example, you lose the ability to produce healthy cartilage. When the cartilage is gone or deteriorated in a joint, the ends of your bones rub together. That's what hurts.

Here's why glucosamine is a vital weapon in the fight against OA.

- It helps produce collagen, which holds your cartilage together.

- It decreases harmful chemical activity that destroys your aging cartilage.

- It helps make your joint cartilage more elastic and shock-absorbing.

Natural glucosamine is made of an amino acid plus glucose — a type of sugar. Most glucosamine supplements are made from the shells of crab, shrimp, and lobster, and sold as glucosamine sulfate. But according to Dr. Jason Theodosakis, author of *The Arthritis Cure*, both forms act the same in your body. Since you're limited to how much glucosamine your body can make, supplements seem a smart decision.

Stop cartilage loss and reduce pain

Many experts say glucosamine is one of the most carefully researched remedies for OA. In fact, 17 major studies have been published since 2000.

One, a well-designed, three-year trial, tested 202 people with osteoarthritis of the knee. Half took 1,500 milligrams of glucosamine sulfate each day; half took a placebo. Remember because these people suffered from OA, they had less cartilage in their knee, and so a smaller gap between the bones. Researchers used X-rays to measure this gap and found those taking the glucosamine regained a tiny amount of joint space each year of the study while the placebo group continued to lose space. That means glucosamine helped save the buffering cartilage in the joint.

> There's more to sex than you think. Like most forms of exercise, sex releases a rush of endorphins, your body's natural painkillers. It also relaxes your muscles and drains tension built up during the day — while keeping your mind off your pain.

In addition, throughout the study, the glucosamine group had less joint pain and stiffness, and no serious side effects from the supplement.

Because of this and other studies, experts in the field believe glucosamine sulfate is the first medicinal treatment that actually slows — perhaps even reverses — the development of OA.

Buy with care

Over 200 glucosamine supplements are available, but Theodosakis says only a few are acceptable. That means many do not contain the ingredients and amounts they claim. Several organizations test and analyze products like glucosamine sulfate supplements, and publish their evaluations. For example, ConsumerLab.com, a private company, offers a subscription service you can access over the Internet at *www.consumerlab.com*.

The Arthritis Foundation recommends these precautions.

- Talk to your doctor before taking glucosamine if you're allergic to shellfish.

- Choose products made by large, well-established companies.

- Read and make sure you understand the ingredient list. Ask your pharmacist for help if necessary.

- Be especially careful if you're already taking a blood-thinner and begin supplementing with a glucosamine-chondroitin combination.

- Always talk to your doctor before taking supplements and never change your prescribed medicine without his advice.

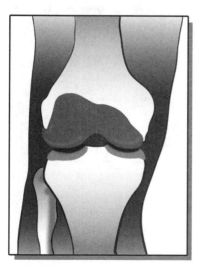

A healthy joint

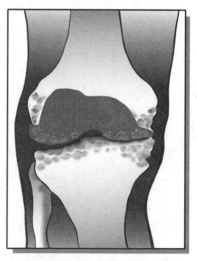

A joint with osteoarthritis

Green tea for allergies

⭐☆☆

Put the brakes on histamine

A tickle, cough, or sneeze could be a reminder you need to brew some tea — green tea. Already famous for being a heart disease and cancer fighter, this popular beverage may be able to claim one more health benefit — taming allergies.

How it works

Scientists think a powerful antioxidant in green tea called methylated epigallocatechin gallate (EGCG) is responsible for its allergy-fighting properties. EGCG interrupts the allergy process by blocking the IgE receptor, which stops your allergic response to outside stimuli, such as dust or pollen. It also prevents the release of histamine, which causes the inflammation associated with allergies.

Earlier studies have shown that similar compounds in green tea may help relieve allergy symptoms, but EGCG appears to be the most potent.

The search for anti-allergens

Unfortunately, no studies on green tea EGCG have yet been done on humans. So far, the research has focused on cells and mice.

If further studies show it works on people, green tea could combat allergens, like dust, pet dander, pollen, and some chemicals. Researchers are also trying to determine how much of it you would have to drink, or if one variety of green tea works better than others.

You'll be the winner if future research supports the green-tea-for-allergies theory. You'll be gaining a simple, inexpensive way to fight annoying allergies. Stay tuned for the latest findings.

Become a green tea expert

You can buy green tea in most grocery and health food stores, either loose or in tea bags. Store it in a dark, airtight container, and keep the container in a cool, dry place. It's best to use green tea within a month or two to reap the most rewards.

Because boiling water destroys some of the antioxidants in green tea, steep it in water that is hot, not boiling, for about three minutes. Drink it before it gets too cool and the tea turns dark brown — a sign the antioxidants are no longer active.

Control allergy triggers

- To kill dust mites and their eggs, wash rugs, bedding, and curtains frequently in hot water, place them outside in the sun for about four hours, or get them dry-cleaned.
- Keep your house as dry as possible to limit the growth of mold.
- During pollen season, keep your windows closed and stay inside.
- Wear a mask to cover your mouth and nose when you garden or clean.
- Shower after being outdoors to remove any pollen clinging to your skin and hair.
- Bathe pets often, treat them with flea repellent, or keep them outside.
- Eliminate soft surfaces in your home — carpets, extra pillows, tablecloths, etc. — and dust often with a wet cloth to trap allergens.
- Drink extra water to control your body's production of histamine, a substance that causes watery eyes and a runny nose.

Green tea for heart disease

★ ★ ★

Stay healthy with flavonoids

Tea is second only to water as the most popular beverage in the world. Many people take a few minutes each day to relax and enjoy a cup of tea. The numbers would be even higher if more folks knew about the extraordinary heart benefits of green tea.

How it works

A number of studies have examined the health benefits of different kinds of tea. Green tea has been found to contain high levels of flavonoids, which are powerful antioxidants. Antioxidants fight harmful molecules called free radicals that scientists think may contribute to heart disease.

Some researchers believe green tea's protective effect may come from its ability to lower blood pressure or LDL cholesterol. Having high blood pressure or high levels of unhealthy cholesterol can increase your risk for heart disease.

Research tells the story

About a decade ago, a study on green tea involving 12,763 men from seven countries looked into how flavonoids in their diet, mainly from green tea, affected their risk of heart disease.

This study found a strong connection between the high flavonoid content of green tea and a lower risk of heart disease. According to the researchers, the more flavonoids you consume, the less likely you are of dying from heart disease.

In its wake came additional studies. Three of them, in particular, highlight green tea's beneficial influence on the heart.

- A two-year study with 393 participants, conducted in Japan, looked into its protective role against heart attacks.

- Another Japanese study, whose main focus was green tea's role in cancer prevention, involved an important sub-study on cardiovascular, or heart and blood vessel, disease.

- The third study, conducted recently in Taiwan, involved 1,507 participants and looked into the relationship between green tea and high blood pressure.

The study on green tea and heart attacks found that those who drank at least one cup of green tea a day were 42 percent less likely to have a heart attack than the people who didn't drink green tea.

The sub-study that focused on green tea's role in preventing cardiovascular disease found that green tea, in terms of heart health, might extend your life. Those who consumed the most green tea lived longer without cardiovascular disease than those who didn't drink green tea.

Eat 'functional foods' every day

Functional foods are foods that provide health benefits beyond basic nutrition. They are important because they contain nutrients that could help reduce the risk of many chronic diseases, like heart disease and cancer.

The FDA divides functional foods into groups. They range from foods whose claims for reducing risk for disease are fully supported by scientific evidence, to foods that have a healthy reputation but lack scientific support for their claims.

Examples of proven functional foods are fruits and vegetables, oat bran, and psyllium. Functional foods needn't be dietary add-ons. Make them part of your normal diet.

In the study of green tea's influence on blood pressure, researchers focused on how long the subjects had been drinking green tea. They concluded that drinking a half-cup (4 ounces) to two-and-a-half-cups (20 ounces) of moderate-strength green tea every day for a year reduced the participants' risk of developing high blood pressure by 46 percent.

Make drinking green tea a habit

You can find green tea in a variety of places, from specialty shops to your local supermarket. Although green tea bags are widely available, you might want to buy your tea fresh.

Look for leaves that have an even color and a delicate, not strong aroma. Since top grades of tea are handpicked, you should see fewer stems in more expensive varieties.

Tea leaves of top grade teas are also more tightly rolled than lower grade teas. This gives the tea a more consistent flavor. It also means a pound of high-quality tea will look smaller than a pound of lower-quality tea.

Green tea for weight loss

Weighing the benefits

Green tea has been used for thousands of years to treat a variety of ailments. Today, this popular beverage is known for fighting cancer and heart and respiratory disease, and many people claim its fat-fighting properties make it a natural complement to any healthy weight-loss program.

How it works

Green tea comes from the same plant that black and oolong teas do. They're just processed differently. Those who love the full-bodied taste of black and oolong teas may be tempted to think the green is too weak. But "weak" probably isn't the right word. Green tea is loaded with potent phytochemicals and antioxidants.

Some studies suggest the antioxidants in green tea, called catechin polyphenols, might help with weight loss by restricting the

Burn extra calories while you play	
Fitness activity	**Calories burned ***
Tennis (singles)	275
Bicycling (no hills)	221
Racquetball	221
Aerobics	203
Badminton (singles)	198
Yoga	180
Tennis (doubles)	171
Ballroom dancing	153
Water aerobics	144
Swing dancing	135
Table tennis	135
Tai chi	135
Golfing (no cart)	131
Strolling	104

* The number of calories a 150-pound person would burn for 30 minutes of activity.

activity of amylase, a carbohydrate-digesting enzyme in saliva. Researchers think this action may slow the digestion of carbo-hydrates, which prevents the sudden rise of insulin in the blood and makes you burn fat instead of storing it. Others suggest the polyphenols in green tea increase your metabolism, helping you burn extra calories.

Extract more effective than brew

In 1985, French researchers conducted one of the first trials on green tea's effect on fat. The study involved 60 middle-age obese women who were put on a diet of 1,800 calories a day and took green tea extract at each meal for 30 days.

After two weeks, the green tea group lost twice as much weight as those on the same diet who took a placebo instead. After four weeks, the green tea group had lost three times as much weight as the placebo group — not to mention significantly greater losses in waist size.

More studies have been done since 1985, but most have focused on how many calories green tea extract burns, which doesn't always mean the same thing as losing weight.

The National Institutes of Health sponsored one of the most recent studies. In this study, 70 moderately obese adults were given two capsules of green tea extract twice a day, containing a daily total of 375 milligrams of catechin.

After three months, their body weight dropped 4.6 percent (that's almost 10 pounds if you began at 200) and 4.48 percent off their waist (2.25 inches if you began at 50 inches).

But here's the catch. You can melt pounds away with green tea, but not by drinking it. You would have to drink an awful lot of green tea to get the dose of fat-burning ingredients the partici-pants in these trials received. They weren't drinking green tea. They were getting large doses of its active ingredients in green tea extract capsules.

Drink to good health

There's no question about it. Green tea's health benefits are amazing. But its usefulness as an aid to weight loss is clearly complementary — it helps. It complements a nutritious diet with limited portions and a daily exercise plan. So don't put your hopes for a dramatic drop in weight in green tea alone.

One more caution — unless the green tea you use is clearly marked "decaffeinated," it will contain caffeine. Although green tea has less caffeine than black tea and about one-third as much as coffee, too much might keep you awake at night or make you feel nervous. If this is true for you, switch to decaffeinated green tea. You can also buy decaffeinated green tea extract.

Guggul for high cholesterol

Herb may harm more than help

Americans spent $1.3 million on guggul supplements in 2002. That's a lot of money to waste.

This highly touted herb has been used medicinally since ancient times. But, when it comes to lowering cholesterol, guggul might be old news.

How it works

Guggul, also known as guggulipid, has an impressive scientific theory on its side.

Researchers believe the active ingredients include plant sterols called guggulsterones. It's easy to remember the specific guggulsterones involved — the E and Z forms.

A better way to cut cholesterol

Slash your cholesterol level by up to 26 percent by adding this to your diet! In a German study, over 200 men participated in a low-fat diet and exercise program, but some also ate oat bran. After just four weeks, the oat bran eaters not only reduced total cholesterol as much as 26 percent, they also cut LDL cholesterol by up to 30 percent. To get these results, the men ate 35 to 50 grams of oat bran daily (about six to eight tablespoons) hidden in breads, sauces, and desserts.

But there's more. Oat bran may protect against colon cancer as well. Beta glucan, a soluble fiber in oat bran, speeds waste products through the large intestine so they have no time to do damage. Beta glucan may also react with tiny organisms to form compounds that protect the colon wall and tame substances that can cause cancer.

Laboratory tests show that both E- and Z-guggulsterones block key hormone receptors involved in cholesterol metabolism. This should lead to more cholesterol being turned into bile acid and less cholesterol being absorbed in the gut.

Guggul boosts bad cholesterol

Unfortunately, theory doesn't always translate into reality. In the first randomized trial in the United States, guggul didn't fare so well.

University of Pennsylvania researchers gave 103 people with high cholesterol either guggul pills or a placebo for eight weeks. Some got a standard dose of 1,000 milligrams (mg) of guggul three times a day, while others took 2,000 mg three times a day.

- Guggul actually raised LDL, or bad cholesterol, by 4 percent in the standard-dose group and by 5 percent in the high-dose group.

- Six people, including five in the high-dose group, even got rashes. The rashes went away once they stopped taking guggul.

- No significant changes took place in total cholesterol, HDL, or triglycerides.

Previous studies in India had shown much more positive results for guggul. But differences in weight and diet between people from India and those from Philadelphia could account for the discrepancies. So could differences in the ways the studies were designed or reported.

Right now, guggul provides more questions than answers. There is certainly not enough evidence to recommend it as a treatment for high cholesterol.

Buyer beware

Besides the troubling results of the Penn study, there are other reasons to be wary of guggul.

You don't always get what you pay for. Four out of five guggul supplements tested by a respected consumer organization contained far less than the expected amount of guggulsterones. One had only 4 percent of what it should.

A study of healthy men showed that when they ate about two-and-a-half cups of beans each day they ate significantly less fat and lowered their total cholesterol levels.

Even if you get a full-strength pill, you might have some unpleasant side effects to contend with. These include rash, nausea, loose stools, vomiting, hiccups, headache, belching, bloating, restlessness, and apprehension.

Fats at a glance

Type of fat	Effect on cholesterol levels	Action plan
Saturated (solid at room temperature) *Sources: Meat, butter, lard, whole milk, cheese, palm kernel oil, coconut oil, chocolate*	Raises both LDL and HDL cholesterol.	Limit to no more than 7 percent of calories daily. Eat lean cuts of meat and use low-fat dairy products.
Polyunsaturated (liquid at room temperature) *Sources: Vegetable oils like corn, safflower, sunflower, sesame, soybean, cottonseed*	Reduces both HDL and LDL cholesterol. Too much may increase cancer risk.	Use oils and soft margarine in moderation, keeping total fat at or below 35 percent of calories per day.
Monounsaturated (liquid at room temperature) *Sources: Olive oil, peanut oil, canola oil, nuts, avocado*	Lowers LDL, HDL stays the same or may be raised in some cases.	Use freely up to 35 percent of total calories per day.
Trans fatty acids (solid at room temperature) *Sources: Margarines, vegetable shortenings*	Raises LDL, lowers HDL.	Reduce or avoid commercially baked products (breads, cookies, cakes) and fried foods from fast-food restaurants. Seek recipes that offer other cooking options.

Guggul may also interact with some prescription drugs, especially statins and those for high blood pressure. If you're taking guggul, make sure you let your doctor know.

Instead of banking on guggul supplements, remember tried and true methods of lowering cholesterol, such as eating a diet low in saturated fat and exercising regularly.

Guided imagery for stress

⭐ ⭐ ⭐

Imagine yourself at peace

Why worry about ending up in the hospital when a 10-minute technique can keep you out of hospitals and save you tons of time and money. In fact, guided imagery may help you worry less about everything.

How it works

Your body has its own emergency response system known as the general adaptation syndrome. When trouble strikes, your adrenaline starts pumping, and your body alerts its stress response so you can react instantly. Next, the body revs up to generate energy, strength, and other resources to help resolve the crisis. After the threat, your body rests and recovers.

But if frequent stress keeps your body on the alert too much, wear-and-tear sets in. Stress may weaken your immune system, raising your risk of health problems. Research has even linked stress to type-2 diabetes, irritable bowel syndrome, cancer, high blood pressure, and heart disease.

Concern about stress's effects on the heart led Dr. Herbert Benson to study the claims of people who practiced meditation.

Soothe stress and more with biofeedback

Here's a simple way to regulate your heart rate, blood pressure, circulation and digestion — and perhaps your stress levels, too. Biofeedback teaches you how to recognize and control changes in your body. It has helped treat conditions ranging from constipation to heart rhythm abnormalities. Biofeedback may also give you power over your physical reaction to stress.

Any gadget that provides information about your body can be a biofeedback device. For example, if you try guided imagery to lower blood pressure and ease stress, a blood pressure cuff can show you which scenes reduce blood pressure. More advanced biofeedback devices may monitor brain waves or measure muscle tension.

You'll need a trained biofeedback specialist and the right equipment to learn to control physical properties like brain waves. But you can teach yourself to monitor your breathing and heart rate — and concentrate on returning them to normal when stress strikes. Relaxation techniques like guided imagery are a good way to start.

He found that blood pressure, heartbeat, and respiration slowed down with meditation.

In fact, he discovered everything that increased with stress, decreased during meditation. Since this was the reverse of the stress response, Benson called these changes "the relaxation response."

But meditation isn't the only road to this relaxed state. Guided imagery can help, too.

Brain scans have shown that visualizing an image triggers the same part of the brain that activates when you look at something. Imagining sounds calls on the brain area used for hearing.

The General Adaptation Syndrome (GAS)

GAS is a theory that describes the body's short-term and long-term reaction to stressors. Hans Selye, a medical doctor and endocrinologist who is sometimes called the "Einstein of Medicine," developed the theory after observing patients with different diseases reacting similarly to the stress of illness.

Phase I "Fight-or-Flight Syndrome" or Alarm Reaction	Phase 2 Resistance	Phase 3 Exhaustion
Adrenal glands produce adrenaline and noradrenaline, which stimulate the heart, liver, kidneys, and lungs.	Brain triggers the release of corticosteroids by the pituitary gland.	Continual use of energy causes physical exhaustion.

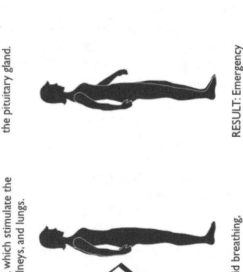

Stressors can be physical, like wounds or surgery, and emotional, like feelings of grief or pressure to perform.

RESULT: Rapid breathing, increased heart rate and blood pressure, increased blood sugar, and muscle tension.

RESULT: Emergency energy is created by the body to handle stress.

RESULT:"Diseases of adaptation" or illness caused or worsened by stress. Colds, flu, arthritis, high blood pressure, and coronary artery disease are just some possibilities.

And daydreaming about the feel of a soft blanket or warm mug perks up the brain centers you'd use while touching those items. Your body responds as if these pleasant events were really happening.

Picture less stress

Researchers recruited 134 open-heart surgery patients to use guided imagery tapes before and after surgery. One week before surgery, the patients began using the tapes several times each day. Hospital staff even helped them listen to the tapes while awaiting anesthesia and during their stay in the recovery area.

On average, the patients' anxiety levels improved by 41 percent after listening to the tapes. They also required a shorter hospital stay than other open-heart surgery patients.

Relaxation techniques, like meditating and guided imagery, might even help keep you out of the doctor's office. Insurance statistics show that meditators require 30 to 87 percent less medical attention than folks who don't meditate. Think of the time and money you can save.

Give guided imagery a try

Guided imagery is a powerful, simple-to-learn technique, but you must practice every day.

- Sit or recline in a comfortable position. Take a few deep, slow breaths and then close your eyes.

- Clench the muscles of your toes to tighten them while you count to 10. Then relax them for a count of 10. Continue up your body, tensing and relaxing each muscle group. By the time you reach the top of your head, the tension in your body should be melting away.

- Imagine a relaxing scene, maybe a deserted beach or a snow-covered mountain. Imagine what you would see, feel, smell, hear, and taste in this place. Become aware of the landscape. If you imagine other people around you, take note of every little thing about them. Pay attention to what you're doing, too. Do this until you feel calm and refreshed.

After you practice a scene regularly, you will be able to recall it during any stressful activity for relief from tension.

Hyaluronic acid for osteoarthritis pain ★★☆

Heal joints naturally

Don't give in to osteoarthritis pain. Fight back with hyaluronic acid (HA), a natural substance produced in your body. Injections or supplements of HA may reduce your pain, lubricate your cartilage, and help your joints glide smoothly over one another.

How it works

Hyaluronic acid is a complex sugar called a mucopolysaccharide that your body produces naturally. It's a thick substance that is part of the synovial fluid. It acts as a lubricant and shock absorber in the cartilage between your joints.

As you age, you produce less hyaluronic acid and have less synovial fluid cushioning your joints, which may lead to the inflammation of osteoarthritis. Studies show that supplementing with HA helps to relieve your painful symptoms.

It's unclear how HA supplements work, but researchers think they may help your body make more hyaluronic acid and affect how your immune cells behave. They also may make the nerves in your joints less sensitive and block substances that promote inflammation.

In the past, you needed to have hyaluronic acid injected directly into your joints, but scientists have developed an oral supplement that shows promise.

Relieves painful joints

The Food and Drug Administration (FDA) approved the use of HA injections for osteoarthritis of the knee in 1997. Researchers are still trying to determine if it works as well for other joint pain.

The FDA has now approved hyaluronic acid for use as a skin filler similar to collagen. When the gel form of HA is injected into your skin, it binds with water, giving your skin volume. HA fills in the wrinkles around your mouth and cheeks, and your wrinkles will disappear for up to four to six months.

A recent study looked at whether a series of HA injections into the big toe would be effective at reducing pain. A group of 47 golfers with osteoarthritis of the big toe received weekly injections of HA for eight weeks. Researchers gathered data on their pain and function for a total of 16 weeks.

At nine weeks, the golfers reported significant improvement in their pain and function, both at rest and while walking on tiptoe. At 16 weeks, the improvements remained, with tiptoe-walking pain significantly reduced.

Oral supplement not proven

Although an oral supplement has been developed, its effectiveness has not yet been proven. An unpublished study by Dr. K. Dean Reeves of the University of Kansas Medical Center focused on the use of HA supplements for treating osteoarthritis knee pain. A dosage of 2 milligrams a day produced a 17-percent reduction in knee pain at two months and a 28-percent reduction at six months.

However, more rigorous scientific studies are needed to support these findings. Although you can buy HA supplements in capsule or tablet form, they are not standardized and may contain other substances. Talk to your doctor first about whether hyaluronic acid is an appropriate treatment for your osteoarthritis pain.

Hypnosis for pain

Ease distress in a unique way

You might not believe in aliens from other planets, but they seem real enough while you're watching Star Wars, ET, or Buck Rogers. Hypnosis may work the same way. In spite of what you know, you might temporarily make yourself believe your pain is easing off.

How it works

When you are hypnotized, you are put into a deeply relaxed state where you are more likely to suspend logic and accept suggestions.

Relieving physical pain is one of the more common uses for this type of therapy, but scientists aren't sure exactly how it works. It doesn't seem to act like drugs on your body's natural painkilling chemicals. Instead, it appears to help keep you focused away from the pain rather than dwelling on it.

Brain wave measurements and images seem to support this theory. Using these tools, scientists have shown that hypnosis activates regions of your brain that control your ability to focus attention.

By concentrating your mind elsewhere, you are aware of your pain but not letting it control your thoughts. This may help you cope with severe pain.

Star of the operating theater

Scientists have been trying to learn whether hypnosis eases pain following surgery. In fact, one review of research found 20 placebo-controlled trials where surgery patients unleashed hypnosis against pain.

The review concluded that hypnosis not only eases pain, it reduces the need for painkillers. However, some health professionals have questioned the soundness of many studies listed in the review.

But the story doesn't end there. Another study found that hypnosis might work against pain during operations where patients aren't usually put to sleep.

This research divided 241 surgery patients into three groups. One group received standard treatment. A second group got unusually attentive treatment from an extra staffer, and the "hypnosis group" received treatment with hypnosis plus the extra attention.

Roll over pain with Beethoven

Listening to music for just 20 minutes a day might tone down pain, a small study suggests. Researchers asked 66 older adults with osteoarthritis pain to participate in a two-week study.

Half the group listened closely to a special classical music tape for 20 minutes each morning. The other half sat in a comfortable place for 20 minutes. By the study's end, the music listeners had significantly less pain. In fact, their pain dwindled throughout the two weeks, while the other participants reported no improvement.

Although this doesn't guarantee music can stop pain for everyone, why not see whether it can work for you? Just be sure to select classical music with a tempo between 60 and 80 beats per minute — and listen closely to the music every day. Who knows? You might get pain relief for a song.

All patients could trigger a dose of pain medicine as often as they wanted. Interestingly, the hypnosis group used lower amounts of painkillers than the group that got standard treatment. The hypnosis group also reported less pain and less anxiety than the other groups.

What's more, the National Institutes of Health may have pegged the pain-fighting potential of hypnosis as far back as 1997. That's when they began funding an eight-year study to find out how hypnosis affects pain and distress from certain cancer-fighting surgeries.

If hypnosis proves successful against surgery pain, it may be effective against other kinds of pain, too. Scientists need to do more research to find out — so stay tuned.

Things to remember

Hypnosis may not work for everyone. According to one estimate, up to 20 percent of people lack the characteristics needed for successful hypnosis. You need a good imagination, the ability to stay focused, trust in the hypnotist, and faith that hypnosis can work.

Hypnotism may be unsafe for people with post-traumatic stress disorder, mental disorders, or those prone to seizures. Other health conditions may also make hypnosis a poor choice for

---

Contact: American Society of Clinical Hypnosis
33 West Grand Avenue — Suite 402
Chicago, IL 60610

American Psychological Association
750 First Street NE
Washington, DC 20002-4242

---

you, so talk with your doctor before you give it a try. And whatever you do, don't substitute pain management for treatment of a serious health condition.

Many people fear they'll end up with a hypnotist who's a con artist or a quack, but qualified, well-trained hypnotists are available. Ask your doctor if he can recommend a properly trained hypnotherapist or write to one of the organizations on the opposite page for referrals.

Low-carbs for weight loss

Long-term effects not known

Atkins-type, low-carb diets have taken dieting by storm. The problem is — besides losing weight, you could lose your health. That's why many nutrition experts are worried.

"Unfortunately," says dietitian Mary Beth Horrell, "they work for quick weight loss. That's what most people want. Even though most of their weight was gained over a period of years, people want to lose it in weeks!"

The anatomy of carbs

Need energy? That's carbs, short for carbohydrates, main role in your body. They're also the most important source of vitamins, minerals, phytochemicals, and fiber.

Yet, as far as nutrition goes, all carbs are not equal. Complex carbs, which include fruits, vegetables, grains, milk, and yogurt, are very important for good health. Simple carbs, or sugars, are less valuable to your health and give all carbs a bad name.

In your quest to cut carbs, it's not wise to limit yourself to the mere 30 grams of daily carbs allowed by these diets. The World Health Organization recommends carbs in the following daily amounts:

- between 50 and 75 percent of your calories (about 200 to 400 grams a day) from complex carbs

- between 27 and 40 grams of fiber

- fewer than 10 percent of your calories from refined sugar sources, like sweets and sweet drinks

Researchers take on Atkins

Atkins is a marketing success — more than 45 million books sold and 20 million followers. But while millions of dollars have been spent promoting the low-carb scheme, nutritionists have been investigating the health facts hidden from us.

A major British medical journal reviewed hundreds of studies on low-carb diets. Three of them, all major randomized trials, have led researchers to conclude:

- People trying to lose weight find it harder to stick with low-carb diets than conventional diets.

- The long-term safety of low-carb diets can't be guaranteed. Many health professionals are worried about an increase in high cholesterol, low blood sugar, colon cancer, and constipation in people following these diets.

- The most solid scientific advice for those who want to lose weight and keep it off is not to radically reduce carbs. It's to cut calories and fat; eat the right combination of foods, like fruits, vegetables, whole grains, and low-fat dairy products; and exercise regularly.

- There's evidence that weight lost on low-carb diets doesn't stay off.

How it works

The low-carb diet's secret to quick weight loss is ketoacidosis. When carbs aren't available for energy, Horrell says, the dieter's body breaks down its own stores of muscle and fat. In the process, compounds called ketones are formed. In order to get rid of these ketones, the body pulls fluid to help wash them out. That's why low-carb dieters have to drink lots of fluids to reduce their risk of dehydration.

Low-carb ketoacidosis isn't lethal, like the type suffered by people with diabetes. "In diabetes, ketones form when there's an absence of insulin, not an absence of carbs. It's very dangerous," says diabetes educator Horrell. "Since people on low-carb diets are still producing insulin, they're not at the same risk as those who have diabetes."

What 10 grams of carbs look like

Low-carb means 30 grams or less of carbohydrates per day. That's about 10 grams per meal. Here's a sampling of what 10 grams (give or take a gram) look like:

- about 3/4 cup of low-fat milk
- 8 ounces whole-milk plain yogurt
- 1/4 cup low-fat vanilla ice cream
- a little less than 1/2 cup of cooked oatmeal
- about 1/4 cup cooked spaghetti
- one extra-thin slice of bread
- one tablespoon cough syrup
- one small banana
- one kiwifruit
- two medium carrots
- 1/5 baked potato
- 1/4 cup prune juice
- 1/3 cup Coke

Ketoacidosis results in loss of water weight, because of the flushing of ketones, and muscle mass, from the breakdown of muscle stores. "These are both losses you don't want," says Horrell.

Beware of "no-think" dieting

Another problem with low-carb dieting is it's not portion-controlled, which is what dieters need. It's too easy. You don't have to think. Just eat protein and fat without limit, and weed out carbs.

"Many of my patients say, 'Just tell me what I can and can't eat.' My answer is always, 'You have to watch *how much* you eat,'" Horrell says.

Horrell concedes two perks in low-carb diets. They can help you realize how much junk you're eating, and they can jumpstart your weight loss program. But don't stay on them for more than a couple of weeks.

Cut out the 'junk' carbs

"I've seen people succeed at weight loss because they limited carbs for a short time, then gradually added them in but continued to control portions," says nutritionist Mary Beth Horrell with Mission Hospital in Asheville, N.C. "They never thought they could eat unlimited quantities of anything."

"The fact is," she says, "most people eat entirely too much carbohydrate. If you cut out the junk — sweets, sweet drinks, white bread — basically carbs with no nutritional value, you'll do great."

"I worked with one patient who cut his carbs down to 60 grams per meal (three meals per day) and lost a ton of weight. We figured that when he'd been going out to eat, he'd get more than 150 grams of carbs in a meal — between hamburger bun, fries, and sweet tea — and he ate out frequently."

"Do something you can do forever," says Horrell. "It's not healthy to limit fruits, whole grains, vegetables, or dairy long term. We've seen the benefits those foods have on blood pressure and heart health."

If you are considering following a low-carb diet, ask your doctor for guidance, especially if you have any health problems.

Lutein for macular degeneration

★★☆

Pigment keeps eyesight sharp

Doctors in ancient Egypt recommended eating liver or applying juice squeezed from cooked liver to the eyes to treat vision problems.

Check out the many benefits you can give your eyes, when you know the secrets contained in this ancient Egyptian prescription.

Most important, liver is chock-full of vitamin A, which does wonders for your vision. But vitamin A, an antioxidant that counters night blindness and cataracts, needs some help.

That's where carotenoids come in. These pigments, which give fruits and vegetables their bright colors, also give your eyes a boost.

Lutein, one of the most important carotenoids, leads the fight against age-related macular degeneration (AMD), the leading cause of blindness for people over 50 in the Western world.

How it works

Lutein, along with fellow carotenoid zeaxanthin, forms the macula, or center, of your eye's retina. With AMD, this area deteriorates, hampering your central vision.

Like Laurel and Hardy or Abbott and Costello, lutein and zeax-anthin make a wonderful team. In fact, you rarely see one mentioned without the other. Together, they go to great lengths to protect your vision.

First, they shield your eyes by filtering out the harmful blue, or ultraviolet, light. They also act as antioxidants to fight tissue damage caused by oxidation, a main factor in macular degeneration.

Future looks bright

Most evidence for lutein is epidemiological. In other words, a higher intake of lutein is associated with a lower risk of AMD in several studies.

For example, in the Multi-Centre Eye Disease Case Control Study, those whose diets contained the most lutein and zeaxanthin had a 57-percent lower risk of developing advanced AMD compared to those who ate the least. However, not all studies support this link.

The Veterans LAST (Lutein Antioxidant Supplementation Trial) study in Illinois showed that lutein, whether taken alone or with other antioxidants, improved macular pigment density and visual function. The one-year study involved 86 men and four women who took a daily dose of 10 milligrams (mg) of lutein.

Eat your greens

How much lutein do you need? Aim for a daily goal of 6 mg per day through your diet. A half-cup of cooked spinach will do the trick.

Other good sources of lutein and zeaxanthin include kale, Swiss chard, collard greens, turnip greens, celery, endive, zucchini, broccoli, lettuce, green peas, melon, guava, oranges, egg yolks, and corn.

You can also find lutein in supplement form, ranging from 6 mg to 25 mg per capsule. Some multivitamins even add .25 mg of lutein. But lutein might not be as effective when taken with other carotenoid supplements.

Keep in mind the long-term safety of lutein supplements has not been proven yet. The optimum dosage also remains unclear. Talk with your doctor before taking supplements.

While lutein supplements may indeed help fend off AMD, the smarter move is to get more lutein and zeaxanthin into your diet. Besides, it's more fun than popping pills — or squirting liver juice into your eye.

Set your sights on saving your vision

- High blood pressure is a risk factor for developing AMD, so monitor your numbers.
- Experts have found a relationship between low levels of zinc and a higher risk of AMD. Get zinc from oysters, crab meat, beefsteak, poultry, enriched cereal, and yogurt.
- The omega-3 fatty acids found in fish like salmon or tuna may protect and restore the cell membranes in your retina.
- Make leafy green vegetables, especially spinach and collard greens, part of your weekly menu. They contain several nutrients vital to eye health.
- Stop smoking and stay away from people who do. Even second-hand smoke can damage your vision.
- Protect your eyes from the sun's ultraviolet rays by wearing sunglasses or a hat.
- Look to brightly colored produce to give your body a dose of antioxidants — natural chemicals that defend your eyes against light damage while supporting the blood vessels to your retina.

⭐ ☆ ☆

Eat your way to stronger bones

What do tomato juice and milk have in common?

They are both important foods for fighting osteoporosis. Milk, of course, provides calcium and is fortified with vitamin D. Tomato juice has lycopene, a nutrient that may also help promote strong bones.

Scientists are crediting good nutrition as an important factor in normal bone growth and the prevention of osteoporosis. One way the nutrients in foods may help protect your bones is by lessening the damaging effects of oxidative stress. Oxidation occurs when unstable molecules called free radicals attack your cells.

Nutrients called antioxidants neutralize the free radicals to protect your cells from harm. Lycopene, a carotenoid found in tomatoes and tomato products, is a powerful antioxidant.

How it works

Your bones are continually changing. Cells called osteoblasts constantly form new bone, while osteoclasts resorb or remove old bone. When you're young, you make new bone tissue faster than you lose it. As you get older, the production process slows down, and you lose bone more quickly than you can replace it. If you haven't built up reserves in your youth, you have a good chance of developing osteoporosis.

Lycopene is an antioxidant that may specifically help keep the bone tearing-down and rebuilding cycle in your favor. In one study, lycopene was shown to positively affect osteoblasts. It stimulated the growth and differentiation of a particular cell called SaOS-2. By aiding the growth of bone cells, lycopene helps your bones get stronger, which in turn helps you fight off osteoporosis.

Bone cells grow faster with lycopene

Researchers at the University of Toronto in Canada studied test-tube cultures of the osteoblast SaOS-2. Lycopene was added at different intervals to some of the cultures, which grew faster than the cultures without lycopene.

Researchers think lycopene's antioxidant qualities helped stimulate the lycopene cultures to grow better, although they say other factors may play a part as well. They hope further research will add tomatoes and lycopene to the arsenal of osteoporosis fighters.

Old advice is still the best

Even with the benefits of lycopene, the best thing you can do for your bones is to get plenty of calcium, vitamin D, and weight-bearing physical activity. The latest Surgeon General's report on osteoporosis says you're never too old or too young to improve your bone health.

It won't hurt to get some extra lycopene, either. In addition to helping your bones, it may help ward off several types of cancer and heart disease. Products made from tomatoes — ketchup, tomato sauce, tomato paste — are your best source. The heating and processing of tomatoes releases more lycopene into your body.

Post-menopausal women are most likely to encounter osteoporosis. One of every two women over 50 will have a broken bone related to osteoporosis in her lifetime. But it strikes men, too. More than 2 million American men have osteoporosis, and millions more are at risk.

So take the Surgeon General's advice — stay active and eat nutritious foods that will help you build strong bones no matter what your stage of life.

Lycopene for prostate cancer

★★☆

Tomatoes pack a powerful punch

It's common knowledge that eating tomatoes can cut your risk of prostate cancer. That's because tomatoes are a good source of lycopene, and lycopene fights prostate cancer, as well as stomach, lung, colon, esophageal, and throat cancers.

In fact, getting plenty of lycopene is a good way to improve your chances to stay healthy and cancer free — without drugs.

How it works

Lycopene is a plant pigment in the carotenoid family that gives tomatoes their brilliant red color. In laboratory tests, this vital nutrient has been shown to fight cancer by slowing the growth of prostate cancer cells.

Some researchers theorize that prostate cancer is related to chronic inflammation. They think it's possible lycopene helps prevent aging cells in the lining of the prostate from oxidizing and becoming damaged during inflammation.

Damage to a cell's DNA can cause it to become cancerous. Although researchers can't be certain, they think lycopene's protective effect comes from its role as a powerful antioxidant that prevents cell damage.

There's more to tomatoes than lycopene

Harvard researchers have found that men who eat at least 10 servings of tomato-based products a week reduce their risk of prostate cancer by 45 percent. A Yale University study showed similar results.

In another study, researchers at Ohio State University wanted to learn if lycopene supplements were as effective as tomatoes at lowering prostate cancer risk.

They took 194 laboratory rats with prostate cancer and divided them into three groups. They fed the control group a balanced diet containing no lycopene. The second group received the balanced diet with added lycopene, and the third group ate the balanced diet mixed with tomato powder (tomato paste with seeds and skins).

Keep your prostate healthy

Whether you want to cut your odds of developing prostate cancer or are looking for natural ways to help your body fight it, don't smoke and try these tips.

- Researchers found that men with the highest blood levels of a form of vitamin E were five times less likely to develop prostate cancer. For more E, eat seed and vegetable oils, nuts, green leafy vegetables, and whole grains.
- Vitamin D may be useful in preventing or treating prostate cancer. But get this nutrient from foods like fortified cereals, not supplements.
- Green tea contains antioxidants called polyphenols that may help protect you from several types of cancer.
- Experts say men who are active are less likely to develop prostate cancer.
- If you gain weight after age 50, you are more likely to get prostate cancer. Talk to your doctor about a healthy weight for you.

At the end of 14 months, the rats that ate the diet containing the tomato powder had a 26- to 32-percent lower risk of dying from the cancer.

The scientists believe additional components of tomatoes combine with lycopene to protect the prostate. They're not exactly sure what's responsible, but they say if you want the health benefits of tomatoes, don't rely on lycopene supplements. Eat tomatoes and tomato products.

Bring on the spaghetti

To help you get the most benefits from tomatoes, keep these things in mind.

- Tomato products, like ketchup and tomato sauce, are more effective than raw tomatoes. Processing and cooking helps break down the cell walls making it easier for your body to absorb the nutrients.

- Carotenoids, like lycopene, are absorbed better when eaten with a little fat.

- Tomatoes mixed with garlic give even more cancer protection, according to researchers in India.

If you're not wild about tomatoes, you can still get lycopene from watermelon, pink grapefruit, guava, papaya, and apricots.

Magnesium for diabetes

Maximize mineral to beat disease

Generations of philosophers have been stumped by one simple question: Which came first, the chicken or the egg?

Scientists studying type-2 diabetes and magnesium deficiency face a similar riddle. Does diabetes cause magnesium deficiency or does magnesium deficiency help cause diabetes?

Whatever the answer, it's important to get enough of this key mineral.

How it works

Evidence shows that diabetics are more likely to be lacking in magnesium. This could be due to increased urination because of abnormal blood sugar levels and the effect of insulin on the body. Diabetes-related kidney disease also may increase magnesium problems.

If you are low in magnesium, you will have a harder time processing carbohydrates, you'll be more open to insulin resistance, and you may suffer high blood pressure, irregular heartbeat and other heart problems, and possibly eye problems. Scientists think you could experience a vicious cycle where diabetes leads to magnesium deficiency, which in turn aggravates your diabetes.

But researchers also think magnesium deficiency may be an important factor in causing diabetes, not just something that affects the progress of the disease. So getting enough magnesium in your diet may help you avoid diabetes as well as keep you healthier if you get it.

More magnesium means less risk

Observational studies of magnesium intake and clinical trials of supplements show that magnesium may help prevent and treat diabetes.

- Harvard researchers tracked 85,060 women for 18 years and 42,872 men for 12 years. Those who got the most magnesium into their diets were one-third less likely to develop diabetes than those who got the least.

- A Simmons College study of 219 women without diabetes showed that women whose diets contained the most magnesium had lower fasting insulin levels than those whose diets had the least. Lower insulin levels mean greater insulin sensitivity, which can reduce the risk of diabetes.

- A Mexican study showed magnesium supplements help diabetics with low magnesium levels. After 16 weeks of taking 2.5 grams of magnesium chloride a day, people in the study boosted the concentration of magnesium in their blood and improved their insulin sensitivity.

In spite of these and other positive studies, it's too early to make a definitive call on magnesium. More clinical trials of magnesium-rich foods and supplements will help.

Eat your way to good health

The Recommended Dietary Allowance (RDA) of magnesium for men 51 years and older is 420 milligrams (mg). For women the same age, the RDA is 320 mg. Unfortunately, many people don't get enough. Intake is especially low among black people.

Foods should provide all the magnesium you need. Good sources of magnesium include avocados, nuts, legumes, whole grains, dark leafy greens, seafood, squash, baked potatoes with skin, broccoli, oatmeal, coffee, tea, and chocolate.

You can also find magnesium supplements in several forms, including magnesium oxide, magnesium gluconate, and magnesium citrate. Supplements range from 64 mg to 500 mg of magnesium per tablet.

Keep in mind that getting your magnesium from supplements may cause diarrhea (magnesium is a common ingredient in laxatives). In fact, diarrhea was one of the side effects reported in the Mexican study of supplemental magnesium. Some people in that study also experienced slight abdominal and bone pain.

Top 3 snacks for extra magnesium		
Snack	**Amount**	**Magnesium**
Trail mix with chocolate chips, salted nuts, and seeds	1 cup	235 milligrams
Pumpkin and squash seed kernels, roasted, with salt added	1 oz. (142 seeds)	151 milligrams
Tropical trail mix	1 cup	134 milligrams

Magnesium may also interfere with the absorption of other minerals, so you might need to add even more supplements to your daily regimen.

We may never unravel the chicken-or-egg riddle, but magnesium's role in diabetes treatment and prevention should someday become clearer. Until then, try adding more magnesium-rich foods to your diet.

Magnets for osteoarthritis pain

Ancient practice gaining status

Using magnets for healing and pain relief is gaining popularity. Yet, despite all the hype, scientific evidence to support the healing power of magnets is skimpy. Although much of the scientific community is skeptical about magnets, clinical research on the subject is just beginning.

How it works

The idea of healing yourself with magnets may sound like a lot of bunk, but scientists suggest some biological reasons why they could possibly work. In simple terms, the magnets may:

- decrease the firing rate of certain neurons, particularly those involved in chronic pain.

- change the activity of certain enzymes that affect inflammation and the creation of free radicals.

- cause minor changes in blood flow.

- regulate the signals within cells.

Researchers say any changes relating to cellular reactions would need strong magnets that could penetrate into deep tissue. If the magnets actually affect the neurons, they would probably need to penetrate only superficially. These are some of the areas that need to be studied before the benefits of magnets can be proven.

Results inconclusive

A recent randomized, double-blind, placebo-controlled study involved 29 people with osteoarthritis pain in their knees. For six weeks, 10 hours a day, half of the study participants wore an active magnetic knee sleeve, while the others wore a placebo magnetic knee sleeve.

Researchers confirmed there was a significant improvement in pain after four hours of closely monitored treatment in the active group, but none in the placebo group. However, at six weeks, there was no difference between the two groups. Both groups had a significant improvement in their pain levels.

At the study's end, 77 percent of the placebo group and 69 percent of the active group believed they were in the group assigned the active magnetic knee sleeve.

This could have been a result of the placebo effect — if you believe something will work, it will. Further studies are needed to determine the effectiveness of magnets on pain relief.

Choose wisely

If you decide to try magnets for your pain, don't just tape that strawberry-shaped magnet that's hanging on your refrigerator to your aching back. The strength of magnets is measured in gauss. The typical refrigerator magnet has about 60 gauss, while most therapeutic magnets have a strength of 300 to 4,000 gauss.

Experts emphasize that more studies are needed to confirm whether magnets work to relieve pain. Although no side effects have been reported from the use of the devices, the possibility that there could be harmful side effects hasn't been ruled out.

Leeches make a comeback

Leeches have been used in medicine throughout most of record-ed history. Yet, like most ancient remedies, they went out of vogue with the arrival of modern surgery and medicines. But now, this ancient medical wonder has finally caught up to science.

Recently, researchers conducted a 91-day study on leech therapy involving 51 patients with osteoarthritis in their knees. Twenty-seven participants used a topical pain reliever twice a day for 28 days, while the other 24 received a single treatment of four to six leeches applied to the painful areas of their knee for about 70 minutes.

The patients undergoing leech therapy experienced a significant reduction in pain starting on the third day. More importantly, their mobility and joint stiffness improved for three months, with just a single application of leeches.

The researchers say leech saliva contains anti-inflammatory substances that can relieve osteoarthritis symptoms. What's more, they hope to develop a pain reliever containing these amazing substances.

Take charge of your osteoarthritis

   Life often involves coping with challenges. If you have arthritis, here are a few ways to meet those challenges head-on.
- Use a rubber grip to make a pen or pencil easier to hold. Ballpoint pens are easier to use than felt-tip pens.
- Raise your bed, so you won't have to bend over when you make it.
- Tuck in your sheets and blankets with a wooden pizza paddle.
- Use a speakerphone in place of a regular telephone.
- Raise the book you're reading to a comfortable height by placing it on several pillows on your lap. Turn the pages with an eraser or a rubber fingertip.
- Glue a small piece of rubber to the underside of your car door handle to make it easier to open.
- Put a webbed lawn chair in your shower stall so you can sit while you bathe.
- Dry off after a shower by putting on a terry cloth bathrobe.

Talk with your doctor before trying this alternative therapy. Magnets can have dangerous side effects if you have certain health conditions, such as pregnancy or wearing a pacemaker.

Margarine substitutes for high cholesterol

★★☆

Cut LDL with a butter knife

A margarine you can spread on your toast that's kind to your heart? It may sound too good to be true, but this margarine actually clobbers artery-clogging cholesterol.

How it works

"Stanols and sterols bind with cholesterol found in food and with bile acids used to make cholesterol in the body," says Lona Sandon, assistant professor of clinical nutrition at The University of Texas Southwestern Medical Center at Dallas. This binding prevents cholesterol from being absorbed into the bloodstream, she says.

Both stanols and sterols come from plants. Sterols from soybeans are the power behind Take Control, a Lipton foods margarine. But a stanol is the secret weapon of Benecol — the competing margarine from Johnson & Johnson subsidiary, McNeil Consumer Products Co. The stanol in canola-based Benecol is a special by-product from the wood processing industry.

Evidence looks strong

You're more likely to have heart disease if you have too much low-density lipoprotein (LDL) cholesterol. That's why LDL is nicknamed "bad" cholesterol. But stanol and sterol margarines can help.

A review of more than 40 research studies concluded that just 2 grams of stanols or sterols daily could help cut LDL cholesterol levels by about 10 percent.

Since increasing your intake to more than 2 grams a day isn't more effective, it's not recommended. However, if you combine these margarines with a low-fat diet or with medications, you might cut LDL by up to 20 percent.

But that's not all. Because the evidence that stanols and sterols help fight heart disease is so strong, the Food and Drug Administration authorized a labeling health claim for sterol- and stanol-powered foods. As long as the foods are low-fat and low-cholesterol, their labels can state they may help slash heart disease risk.

Although stanol and sterol margarines are generally recognized as safe, the products haven't been around long enough for long-term safety studies.

Here's the scoop

Stanol and sterol margarines are most helpful if your cholesterol is only modestly high — around 200 to 239 mg/dL.

"The most benefit seems to come with about 2 grams per day of the plant stanol/sterol — or using 1 tablespoon of the spread, two to three times per day while following a healthy diet and exercise plan," says Sandon.

To get maximum mileage from your margarine, use it to replace fats you normally eat. Otherwise, you'll gain weight and cancel out the spread's benefits.

Eat colorful fruits and vegetables to help control weight and prevent nutrient losses. "These margarines may lower carotenoid levels in the blood by 10 to 20 percent," Sandon says. But you can fix that. "Just one extra serving of a carotenoid-rich fruit or vegetable — such as carrots, sweet potato, pumpkin, tomatoes, apricots, or spinach — has been shown to prevent any lowering of carotene levels," Sandon says.

Eating cholesterol in foods doesn't increase your blood cholesterol as much as eating saturated fats. Foods high in saturated fat include meat, egg yolks, whole milk, cheese, butter, as well as a few vegetable fats, like coconut oil, palm oil, and hydrogenated vegetable shortenings.

Don't use these margarines to replace your medication. Although the spreads work well with medicines, like statins, they're no substitute.

Look for cholesterol-cutting margarine in your grocery store. If you plan to use the margarine for cooking or want zero trans-fats, check the labels. "Some versions of the

Cholesterol guidelines	
Less than 200 mg/dL	Desirable
200-239 mg/dL	Borderline high
240 mg/dL and above	High

products are trans-fat free, which means they contain less than 0.5 grams of trans-fat per serving.

The regular stanol margarines that can be used for baking and cooking contain less than 1 gram of trans-fat per serving," says Sandon. "The amount of trans-fat is no more, maybe even less, than one would find in a typical margarine."

Talk with your doctor before trying sterol or stanol margarines, especially if you take cyclosporine or similar medications.

Meal replacements for weight loss ★★☆

Slim down with bars and shakes

Meals packaged like candy bars or milkshakes are tasty and convenient, but do they really help you lose weight? Some researchers think so. Although they'll never be a match for nutritious meals, they might be worth a try.

How it works

Eating a meal-replacement product, either in liquid or solid form, is a popular way to cut calories and lose weight. Many food bars are geared toward people on a particular weight loss plan. They do offer certain advantages, like giving you a specific portion size and providing a convenient way to eat if you would skip a meal otherwise.

This might help keep you from getting too hungry and overeating later. A recent study found that certain meal-replacement products reduced hunger and the desire to eat for five hours following consumption.

Those who promote certain diet plans also claim that by eating low- or moderate-carbohydrate foods, the insulin level in your blood won't rise as much after meals, which may help you burn more fat and lose weight. But studies have found these bars don't reduce insulin levels as much as expected.

Results were impressive

University of Kentucky researchers examined the results of four studies on meal-replacement bars and shakes involving 470 women and 133 men. The participants were encouraged to use meal-replacement products twice a day for six months.

At the end of the study, the average female participant lost 9.3 percent of her initial body weight, or about 17 pounds. The average male participant lost 8.6 percent, or about 19 pounds.

The research also found that meal replacements demand less intervention than other weight loss plans. That means fewer hours of weight loss instruction and fewer visits to the doctor or diet counselor.

Researchers concluded that meal replacements are effective weight loss tools. Just remember — your success depends on the number of calories you consume and your faithfulness to the diet plan.

Ask for advice

One dilemma dieters face is the huge variety of available products. A grocery store's nutrition section can be bewildering. There are shakes and bars for energy, protein, diet, and meal replacement.

And to make matters worse, you have to choose among "energy-restricted," "low-carb," and "very-low-carb" products. The differences aren't always clear.

Do some research before you shop so you'll know what to look for. You could also ask your doctor or nutritionist for advice. In addition, don't overlook some of these products' known shortcomings.

- Their nutrition labels are known to be suspect, sometimes underreporting carbohydrates, saturated fat, and sodium.

- They're very low in dietary fiber, which is important for good health.

- They may contain ingredients you don't want, like herbs or stimulants, like caffeine.

Be sensible and keep this in mind — the best way to lose weight is to burn more calories than you take in by practicing portion control and getting regular physical activity.

Melatonin for insomnia

★★★

Prime your body for sleep

Few things are more frustrating than lying in bed for hours and not being able to sleep. Except maybe waking an hour before your alarm goes off and staring at the ceiling with no hope of getting more rest.

Having insomnia is not just an unpleasant experience. It can result in serious health problems, like depression, breathing abnormalities, and heart disease.

How it works

Melatonin is a hormone produced by the pineal gland located at the base of your brain. It regulates your body clock's natural wake-sleep cycle, which is known as circadian rhythm. Your body produces low amounts of this hormone during the day while you're exposed to bright light, and more at the end of the day as it gets darker. The higher amounts at night prepare your body to fall asleep.

Because it plays a pivotal role in the natural sleep cycle, researchers think melatonin may help people with sleep problems, particularly

Beware of sleep-robbing drugs

Several types of drugs can cause insomnia. These are the most common:
- antihypertensives
- beta-blockers
- corticosteroids
- decongestants
- diuretics
- Levodopa
- oral contraceptives
- phenytoin (Dilantin)
- stimulants
- thyroid hormone
- selective serotonin reuptake inhibitors

If you suspect a drug you are taking is interfering with your sleep, talk with your doctor about switching to another medication or lowering the dosage. Don't stop taking the drug without his approval.

older adults. It's believed that melatonin levels tend to drop as you get older, although some recent research has not supported this. By using supplements to increase your body's natural supply, you may get a better night's sleep.

Supported by research

An Israeli study showed melatonin replacement therapy may improve sleep quality for some insomnia patients. In the five-week study, 372 insomniacs over age 55 were treated for two weeks with a placebo and for three weeks with 2 milligrams per night of melatonin.

Researchers looked at how much melatonin participants excreted. They found that 30 percent, or 112 patients, expelled lower than normal levels of the hormone. These 112 patients also benefited significantly from the replacement therapy as compared with participants who excreted higher amounts of melatonin.

Researchers concluded that a low nightly production of melatonin was associated with insomnia in older adults. They also believed this low melatonin production could help identify people who might benefit from melatonin replacement therapy.

Consider these problems

If you're considering taking melatonin to help you sleep at night, consult your doctor first. If you have asthma, he may advise against it. Research has shown melatonin may promote inflammation. Many asthmatics find their problems increase at night, and it's possible melatonin may be a contributing factor.

Melatonin is generally safe for short-term use, but be aware of these other possible problems.

- Drowsiness, impaired mental alertness, and loss of balance are common, so don't drive or operate heavy machinery for several hours after use.

- It may affect testosterone levels and impair sperm function in men.

- High doses can prevent ovulation in women.

- It may weaken insulin action in diabetics.

- You shouldn't take it if you use tranquilizers, sedatives, antidepressants, or if you have lupus, a hormonal imbalance, autoimmune disease, or rheumatoid arthritis.

Be a smart consumer

You can buy several different kinds of melatonin pills. The fast-release kind will get into your bloodstream quicker, and the slow-release pills will keep the hormone at a more even level throughout the night. One kind may help you sleep better than the others, so you may want to experiment.

You can increase your melatonin naturally by changing what you eat, experts say. Start eating more whole grains, legumes, nuts, milk, meat, fish, poultry, and eggs. These foods don't contain melatonin, but they contain the amino acid tryptophan. The body converts tryptophan into serotonin and finally to melatonin. Eating any of these foods about an hour before bedtime may increase your melatonin and help you sleep better.

You can also eat foods that contain melatonin — like oats, sweet corn, rice, ginger, cherries, tomatoes, bananas, and barley.

Other ways to increase your melatonin levels naturally:

- Keep your bedroom very dark.
- Get eight hours of sleep every night.
- Get plenty of sunshine during the day.

Melatonin for migraines

☆ ☆ ☆

Combat headaches with amazing hormone

The intense throbbing, pressure, and pain of a migraine can drive you straight to bed. If you're like millions of others who can barely function when one hits, you'll welcome a new way to fight back. The hormone melatonin shows promise for migraine relief and just may help you knock them out of the ring.

How it works

Scientists have several theories as to why migraine headaches occur. One explanation is that they result from an irregularity in the pineal gland located at the base of your brain. This gland produces melatonin, and research has found that migraine sufferers tend to be low in this critical hormone.

Migraineurs are also bothered by environmental factors such as light, noise, temperature, smell, and humidity. Some researchers suggest the pineal gland is the connection between environmental triggers and migraine headaches.

If you have sleep problems in addition to migraines, melatonin may be the key to relief. Melatonin regulates your sleep-wake cycle. If your normal cycle is out of sync, you may be more susceptible to migraines and other types of headaches. By bringing your natural cycle back to normal,

Scent can be a powerful healer. That's why aromatherapy often works against the pain and discomfort of migraines. Try gently rubbing a single drop of rosemary, lavender, or chamomile essential oil onto your skin where it hurts the most. Or try just a sniff of peppermint oil. Some say it is as effective as acetaminophen in reducing head pain.

221

melatonin supplements may help prevent migraines from occurring. Several studies have found that giving melatonin to migraine sufferers helped to relieve pain and prevent a recurrence in some cases.

Increase melatonin, decrease migraines

Researchers recently conducted a small study using 34 migraine sufferers, with and without aura, who experienced two to eight migraines a month. During the three-month study period, patients took 3 milligrams (mg) of melatonin 30 minutes before bedtime every night.

Remarkably, at the end of the study, 25 percent of the participants reported suffering no migraines. Roughly 22 percent had 75 percent fewer migraines. In addition, 31 percent experienced a reduction between 50 and 75 percent. Plus, melatonin therapy lowered their headache intensity and duration and decreased their use of painkillers and medication.

> Ginger might help lessen the agony of a migraine attack as well as the nausea that often comes with it. Herbalists generally recommend 2 to 4 grams of ginger a day, but you may need more. Look for ginger root in the produce section of your supermarket, or buy supplements as gelatin capsules. Add it to your diet gradually.

Researchers were encouraged by the results and recommended studies be done testing melatonin against a placebo.

Don't overdo it

Since migraine studies are still preliminary, a recommended dosage has not been established and will vary for each person. Your body only requires about 0.3 mg of this hormone a day, so start off slow and don't go over 1 mg daily without the guidance of your doctor. Because it is a hormone, researchers are not sure how long-term use of melatonin may affect your body.

Veto migraines with prevention tips

Don't let painful migraines run your life. Stop them before they start with these natural remedies that have helped people just like you.

- Discover if there are any specific foods that trigger your migraines — and avoid them. Common culprits are cheese, red wine, chocolate, and wheat.
- Some experts think a magnesium deficiency could cause painful migraines. Talk to your doctor about supplements or get this nutrient naturally from brown rice, popcorn, broccoli, green peas, potatoes, shrimp, clams, and skim milk.
- Try a 30-minute head and neck massage several times a week. It may reduce the number of migraines you experience.
- Omega-3 fatty acids can reduce the number and intensity of migraines. Natural sources are tuna, cod, salmon, and flaxseed.
- Postmenopausal women with migraines could benefit from a combination of calcium and vitamin D. Get this therapy in one gulp by drinking fortified low-fat or fat-free milk.

You can purchase melatonin supplements in tablets or capsules at your local pharmacy. They come in time-release and quick-release forms to treat various types of insomnia. Ask your doctor which is better for your migraines. Also, check with your doctor about interactions with other medications you take, especially NSAIDs, beta-blockers, antidepressants, diuretics, and vitamin B-12. Avoid alcohol or caffeine while taking melatonin.

Rather than take a supplement, you can increase your melatonin levels naturally with foods like oats, sweet corn, and rice. Cherries are an extra rich source of melatonin, so give yourself a sweet treat, and eat a handful right before going to bed. They may be just what you need to ward off the nightmare of another migraine.

Mental exercise for memory loss

★★★

Mind games mend your memory

Your brain may not be a muscle, but the same rule applies — use it or lose it. Challenge your mind regularly, and you strengthen it against memory loss. Let it get lazy, and you risk losing the mental sharpness you need to live independently.

How it works

You lose hundreds of thousands of precious brain cells every day. That's not science — it's science fiction. You only lose a lot of neurons, or brain cells, when you suffer from a stroke, Alzheimer's disease, or other major disorder.

Otherwise, not many neurons actually die. Some of them just shrink. That's partly why your mind seems to slow down and forget things, a condition known as age-associated memory impairment. It may sound serious, but it doesn't have to be permanent.

Promising studies show reading, doing crossword puzzles, and even listening to music may hold the secret to staying mentally alert as you age. Challenging leisure activities like these stimulate your brain the way a workout invigorates your body. The result — a memory that's as sharp as a tack at any age.

Mental exercise seems to have three major biological effects.

- builds new neurons
- creates new connections, or synapses, between neurons
- fortifies existing synapses

In other words, mental workouts strengthen your brain and help it grow, not just grow older.

Here's another benefit. By increasing the number of cells and connections in your brain, some scientists think you build up a savings account of extra neurons and synapses, called cognitive reserve, that shore you up against mental decline later in life.

Challenge your mind to keep it sharp

A number of studies show that mentally active people tend to test higher in their cognitive, or thinking, abilities and begin old age with better thinking skills.

The most convincing recent research comes from the Rush Medical Center in Chicago where scientists studied more than 4,000 older adults for an average of five years. In the beginning, the people took thinking tests and answered questions about their leisure activities. Every three years, they tested again. In the end, those who participated in the most mind-challenging activities suffered the least mental decline — 35 percent less than their peers.

Walk away from forgetfulness

Heart-healthy exercises may strengthen your mind as well as your body.

Researchers at the University of Illinois divided older adults into two groups — one began a walking program, the other a stretching program. In just six months, the walking group not only improved their physical fitness, they also outperformed the stretching group in tests of thinking skills.

These scientists say that walking and other moderate cardiovascular exercises, which increase your heart rate and get your blood moving, can improve your mental fitness and enhance your quality of life. Other research suggests that listening to music, particularly classical music, while you exercise could boost your brain power even more.

Bored with the same old brain games? Give yourself new challenges with online puzzles. Web sites such as *www.AllStarPuzzles.com* and *www.RinkWorks.com/brainfood* offer all the mind-benders you can handle, including cryptograms, memory games, and logic problems, for free.

You may even live longer thanks to mental exercise, besides keep your brain sharp well into your 90s. While studying an order of Catholic nuns called the Sisters of Mankato, scientists discovered that nuns who taught, studied, or performed other challenging mental tasks lived longer than those who did mostly physical labor.

Just feeling confident in your mental abilities may help you remember more. Researchers in another study found that people's memory depended largely on their attitude toward aging. Those who didn't expect to become forgetful or mentally slow with age had better memories than people who bought into old-age stereotypes. Some of these youthful thinkers even scored as well on memory tests as younger adults.

Super ways to jog your memory

So how much "exercise" do you need to stay fit? Studies suggest the more, the better. You don't have to read encyclopedias to get a good mental workout, either. The kinds of brain-boosting activities scientists cite most are as simple as playing bridge and doing crossword puzzles — essentially, anything that makes you think.

Mental exercises are natural, proven remedies for improving your memory. Try these super ways to slow and even reverse the aging process.

- read or work crossword puzzles
- play chess, cards, or board games
- dance and listen to music
- play a musical instrument

Memory-stealing prescription drugs

Your medication might be making off with your memories. Check this list of popular drugs. Talk with your doctor about changing your prescription if you think one is causing memory loss.

Condition	Generic drug	Brand name
High blood pressure	Atenolol	Tenormin, Tenoretic
	Bisoprolol fumarate and Hydrochlorothiazide	Ziac
	Fosinopril sodium	Monopril
	Lisinopril	Zestril, Prinivil
	Lisinopril and Hydrochlorothiazide	Zestoretic, Prinzide
	Losartan potassium	Cozaar
	Losartan potassium-hydrochlorothiazide	Hyzaar
	Metoprolol succinate	Toprol-XL
	Propranolol hydrochloride	Inderal, Inderide
Heart disease or High cholesterol	Fluvastatin sodium	Lescol
	Pravastatin sodium	Pravachol
	Simvastatin	Zocor
Anxiety or Depression	Alprazolam	Xanax
	Bupropion hydrochloride	Wellbutrin
	Lorazepam	Ativan
	Nefazodone hydrochloride	Serzone
Sleeping disorders	Triazolam	Halcion
	Zolpidem tartrate	Ambien

- visit a museum or head to the theater
- get involved in clubs and other social groups
- volunteer your time
- sign up for a local college course

Start this effective journey now, and you'll improve and prevent the loss of your memory. Vary your activities so you work different brain cells every day to reap the most benefit.

Nasal sprays for sinusitis

★★☆

Relief for irritating symptoms

Sinusitis is more than a stuffy nose. It's an inflammation or infection of your sinuses that can cause a dull throb behind your eyebrows, pain in your cheeks and teeth, and a low-grade fever.

Acute sinusitis lasts for three weeks or less. Chronic sinusitis usually lasts for three to eight weeks, but it can stay with you for months or years.

Every year, about 37 million Americans get sinusitis. Because the causes vary from one person to the next, effective treatments vary, too.

How it works

Sinuses are hollow air spaces. You have four pairs of sinuses, called the paranasal sinuses, located around your nose and eyes. Each sinus has an opening into your nose so air and mucus can be exchanged.

Colds, allergies, and weather changes can trigger sinusitis. Because the sinuses and nostrils share the same membrane,

---

Baby your sinuses when infection strikes

In many cases of sinusitis, antibiotics are the only way to end your misery. But your doctor may also prescribe steroid nasal sprays, oral steroids, decongestants, and pain relievers. Follow usage directions carefully. If you take certain medications too long or stop them too early, you can do more harm than good.

Home remedies cannot cure a sinus infection, but they might make you feel better.

- Run a vaporizer or sit in a steamy shower.
- Apply moist heat to painful areas of your face.
- Sip a hot drink.

Try to prevent chronic sinus attacks by avoiding cigarette smoke and other irritants, running a humidifier in your home, and installing electrostatic filters in your heating and cooling units.

---

anything that stuffs up your nose can also stuff up your sinuses. When sinuses can't drain, they breed bacteria, which can complicate sinusitis.

If your sinuses are infected, your doctor will probably prescribe an antibiotic. Nasal sprays, including saline solutions, decongestants, steroids, and antifungals, help keep the sinuses open and relieve symptoms.

- saline nasal spray — a salt water spray you can buy at any drugstore. It loosens and rinses away mucus and moistens dry membranes.

- decongestant spray — an over-the-counter spray that temporarily unblocks sinus openings and reduces nasal congestion. Afrin and Neo-Synephrine are two of the better-known brands.

- steroid spray — reduces inflammation and mucous production in chronic sinusitis. It does not provide immediate relief and may require several weeks of regular use to be effective. Rhinocort, Nasacort, and Flonase are steroid sprays.

- antifungal spray — used to treat chronic sinusitis triggered by a fungus.

Unfortunately, research has found that 10 to 25 percent of sinusitis victims continue to have symptoms, even with the help of nasal sprays and antibiotics.

Choose the right spray for the job

Saline sprays are safe for everyone, not addictive, and can be used as often and for as long as needed. Curiously, they haven't received much attention from researchers. Nevertheless, they receive "honorable mention" in studies about other types of nasal sprays.

Evidence doesn't support decongestant sprays as a lasting treatment for sinusitis. They will reduce sinus inflammation for a few hours but shouldn't be used for more than three days at a stretch. Overuse results in rebound — congestion returning with a vengeance once you stop using them. And don't be surprised if these sprays make your nose run, sting, or itch.

Don't use decongestants if you have heart disease, high blood pressure, thyroid problems, diabetes, or an enlarged prostate without your doctor's consent.

Steroid sprays, also called corticosteroids, are designed to treat indoor and outdoor allergies. Since most acute sinusitis isn't caused by allergies, it's not surprising that clinical trials on acute sinusitis haven't found steroid sprays to be very effective. If you have chronic sinusitis, your doctor might suggest using a steroid spray every day.

Clinical trials show that antifungal sprays might help if your immune system overreacts to common airborne funguses. The degree to which funguses contribute to sinusitis is still up for debate. Some researchers think most sinusitis is a reaction to funguses, while others believe they only affect a certain group of people.

Over-the-counter and prescription nasal sprays can help treat the symptoms of sinusitis but only as a complement to antibiotics, surgery, or other treatments prescribed by your doctor.

Nasal strips for snoring

★★☆

Breathe easier all night

Snoring not only affects your sleep — and anyone else's within earshot — it can affect your health as well. High blood sure, artery disease, muscle fatigue, and chronic heada some of the conditions that can result.

But take heart. If your snoring isn't c̲ by a serious problem, finding relief may be as simpl cky strip across your nose.

How it works

When you're asleep and your airways are blocked, you snore. It can be caused by the vibration of your soft palate or air passing through blocked or swollen nasal passages. Plenty of remedies exist — some work, some don't. But one drug- and surgery-free snoring solution is gaining acclaim — nasal strips.

Their simplicity makes nasal strips a brilliant invention. They are just strips of flexible plastic with an adhesive backing. When you stick them across your nose just beneath the bridge, they automatically try to straighten. This creates a gentle, continuous pressure that makes the nostrils expand. And voila! The nasal airways open, airflow improves, and the frequency of snoring drops.

Helps you sleep better

A small European study involving habitual snorers with confirmed nasal obstructions but no sleep apnea put the Breathe Right brand of nasal strips to the test.

Compared to a placebo, the strips significantly reduced the amount — but not the loudness — of snoring in the 12 participants. Researchers speculated that the sound was unaffected because it is created in the throat, not the nose.

Easy strategies to silence the snoring

Surf the drugstore aisles or the Internet and you'll find oodles of snore "cures." Some might work for you or your wood-sawing spouse. Many don't. Before you plunk down the cash for the latest strip, spray, or strap, try these natural remedies.

- Lose weight. Carrying extra pounds means more soft tissue around your throat. This can block your air passages.
- Be aware of side effects. Anything that works as a sedative, like alcohol or some antihistamines, causes your tissues to relax and can contribute to snoring.
- Stop smoking.
- Don't sleep on your back. Sew a tennis ball into the back of your nightclothes to make you roll over.
- Elevate your head to breathe easier. Propping up the whole upper part of your bed works better than adding extra pillows.

Snoring is often a symptom of sleep apnea. Talk to your doctor about this serious condition that is widely undiagnosed.

Buying advice

A nasal strip may be just the thing to relieve your snoring and give you a more comfortable night's sleep. But you need to use it correctly. First of all, make sure you get the right size. You need a strip that only covers your nose — it's too big if it touches your cheeks. Then follow the directions to make sure you place it in the right spot.

Since nasal strips are disposable and can be used only once, you may want to save money and buy generic rather than name brands.

If nasal strips and other self-help remedies don't work, make sure you see a doctor about your snoring. It may be a symptom of a more serious health issue that you can't afford to overlook. And you may need more radical measures to overcome your problem, such as apnea treatment or weight loss.

> If you snore, you share a trait with some illustrious company — Abe Lincoln, Franklin Roosevelt, Winston Churchill, and Benito Mussolini, to name a few. Snorers like Melvin Switzer, Kare Walkert, and Mark Hebbard rank among the world's loudest, with snores of 90 decibels or better — as loud as a firetruck siren.

Nuts for heart disease

Grab heart help by the handful

Money may not grow on trees but heart protection can. Tree nuts such as walnuts and almonds may help defend your heart — and you can call in tasty peanuts for reinforcements.

How it works

Nuts may be high-fat foods, but they're cholesterol-free, and most are low in the saturated fats that send cholesterol skyward. Nuts are also high in monounsaturated and polyunsaturated fats — the ones that reduce cholesterol.

In addition, most nuts serve up arginine. Your body uses this amino acid to produce a substance that fights plaque buildup in your arteries. Another amino acid, homocysteine, can damage arteries if too much piles up in your blood, but the folic acid in many nuts can help prevent that.

Soluble fiber in nuts may cut LDL cholesterol, and many nuts provide heart-healthy minerals like copper and magnesium. Phytosterols in nuts may help your heart, too.

Nuts are also rich in vitamin E, but the U.S. Preventive Services Task Force has concluded that scientists haven't got

---

Add 10 extra years to your life

Researchers from Loma Linda University tracked more than 34,000 Seventh-Day Adventists for 12 years. They found that Adventist men can expect to live more than seven years longer than the average Californian, while Adventist women can tack on an extra four-and-a-half years.

Of course, not all Adventists live perfectly healthy lives. But an Adventist who eats a vegetarian diet, exercises regularly, eats nuts more than five times a week, maintains a healthy weight, and doesn't smoke will live about 10 years longer than an Adventist who does none of those things.

There's no reason why the Seventh-Day Adventists in California should be the only ones to benefit from their healthy lifestyle. You can add an extra 10 years to your life by following their healthy lifestyle. It's the most powerful treatment for reducing your risk of heart attack and stroke and improving the quality of your life.

enough evidence to determine whether vitamin E helps prevent heart disease.

Scientists think omega-3 fatty acids may pitch in to avert the irregular heartbeat that can cause "sudden death" — death within an hour of a heart attack. Walnuts are a good source of an omega-3 called alpha-linolenic acid or ALA. Other nuts have ALA in smaller amounts.

Crack down on heart risks

Several studies suggest that nuts help prevent heart trouble.

Different nuts may help your heart in different ways. Small studies hint that almonds, pecans, walnuts, and macadamias may trim cholesterol. Pistachios lead all other nuts in potassium — a mineral that eases blood pressure. And peanuts contain resveratrol, a plant estrogen that works like an antioxidant to combat heart disease.

- Researchers studying 30,000 Seventh Day Adventists found that those who ate nuts at least five times a week reduced their risk of heart attack by 50 percent, compared to those who ate them less than once a week.

- A study of 40,000 postmenopausal women also found a lower risk of heart disease among frequent nut eaters.

- A 17-year study of 21,000 male doctors suggested the odds of death from heart disease were 30 percent lower in men who ate nuts at least twice a week. Compared to those eating nuts less often, men who ate two or more 1-ounce servings of nuts weekly had 47 percent less risk of sudden death.

Moreover, the Food and Drug Administration (FDA) recently approved a health claim for labels of whole or chopped walnuts. The claim says that "supportive but not conclusive research" shows that eating 1.5 ounces of walnuts daily may reduce heart disease risk — but only if the nuts don't boost calorie intake and are part of a low-cholesterol, low-saturated-fat diet.

Nuts: A Handful of Nutrition

Nuts	Nuts per 1 ounce serving	Calories	Protein (grams)	Fat				Omega-6 fatty acids (grams)	Omega-3 fatty acids (grams)	Vitamin K (mcg)[1]	Vitamin E or alpha-tocopherol (mg)[2]	Phytosterols[3] (mg)	Beta carotene (mcg)	Lutein + zeaxanthin[4]
				Total	Sat	Mono	Poly							
Almonds	24 nuts	160	6	14	1	9	3	3	0	0	7.3	34	.9	.3
Brazils	6-8 nuts	190	4	19	5	7	7	6.8	.02	0	1.6	n/a	0	0
Cashews (dry roasted)	18 nuts	160	4	13	3	8	2	2.2	.05	10	.3	45	0	6.5
Hazelnuts	20 nuts	180	4	17	1.5	13	2	2.2	.02	4	4.3	27	3.1	26.1
Macadamia (dry roasted)	10-12 nuts	200	2	22	3	17	.5	.4	.06	n/a	.2	32	0	n/a
Peanuts	28 nuts	170	7	14	2	7	5	4.4	0	0	2	n/a	0	0
Pecans	20 halves	200	3	20	2	12	6	5.9	.28	1	.4	29	8.2	4.8
Pine nuts (pignolias)	157	190	4	20	2	6	10	9.4	.05	15.3	2.6	40	4.8	2.6
Pistachios (dry roasted)	49 nuts	160	6	13	1.5	7	4	3.9	.07	3.7	.6	61	44	341.6
Walnuts	14 halves	190	4	18	1.5	2.5	13	10.8	2.6	.8	.2	20	3.4	2.6

1 mcg = micrograms
2 mg = milligrams
3 phytosterols have shown cholesterol-lowering activity
4 Some studies have shown a relationship between higher intake of lutein and a lower risk of eye diseases.
Source: USDA National Nutrient Database for Standard Reference, Release 16, 2003.

The FDA is considering a similarly worded claim for most other nuts. But cashews, macadamias, Brazil nuts, and some pine nut varieties won't ever display the claim because they have too much saturated fat.

Be a health nut

Take the FDA's advice. Don't just add nuts to your diet. Eat them in place of other high-calorie foods. Otherwise, the fats and calories in nuts may lead to weight gain. A review of nut research found that nut eaters don't have a higher body mass index than folks who don't eat nuts — as long as the nuts replace another high-calorie food in the diet.

Studies suggest 1 to 2 ounces of nuts a day — about a handful — may be enough to do your heart good. Sample almonds, walnuts, peanuts, pecans, chestnuts, hazelnuts (filberts), pistachios, and more. Just try to avoid nuts coated with candy, sugar, honey, or salt. If you're salt-sensitive, check the label for sodium content.

Nuts are a common cause of food allergies. Call for emergency help if you experience any of these symptoms within an hour of eating nuts — skin rash, scratchy or swollen throat, stuffy or runny nose, sneezing, difficulty breathing, stomach upset, vomiting, diarrhea, or bloating.

Omega-3 fatty acids for cancer

Tackle risk with more than fish

You may have heard that omega-3 fatty acids can help you resist cancer, but there's more to the story.

How it works

Omega-3 fatty acids are polyunsaturated fats your body can't make on its own. You get them from delicious cold-water fish and some seeds and nuts. But omega-3s may be hampered by a hidden rival — the omega-6 fatty acids lurking in vegetable oils, fried foods, meats, eggs, milk, processed grains, and anything containing corn or soybean oils.

When you take in either omega-3s or omega-6s, your body breaks them down into other substances. Several by-products created from omega-6 fatty acids are thought to have cancer-promoting effects, explains Paul Terry Ph.D., assistant professor of epidemiology at Emory University. "In contrast, the by-products of omega-3 fatty acids are thought to help prevent or retard the development of certain forms of cancer," he says.

Not surprisingly, studies suggest that most of us rack up 10 to 25 times more omega-6s in our diets than omega-3s. That could provide countless opportunities for carcinogens, or cancer-causing substances, to form.

But omega-6s can't create their cancer-building by-products without help from enzymes — the same enzymes omega-3s need to create cancer-fighting chemicals. So anytime both fatty acids show up, the battle for the enzymes is on.

"Because omega-3 fatty acids usually compete for these enzymes successfully, the higher the ratio of omega-3 to omega-6 fatty acids the better," says Terry. For most of us, that means adding more omega-3s, while subtracting omega-6s.

Changing proportion shows promise

Terry and his colleagues recently reviewed the research that examined whether omega-3s can help prevent hormone-related cancers, like breast and prostate cancer. Here's what they found. Although there is compelling evidence from test tube studies and animal experiments, research with humans has yet to establish a strong case for eating fish to reduce risk of these cancers.

How to get more omega-3

For your best sources of omega-3, check this chart. Portions are based on an uncooked serving size of 100 grams — approximately 3 to 3 1/2 ounces.

Food	Omega-3 in grams	% Omega-3 in total fat	Total fat in grams
Sardines in oil	3.3	21	15.5
Pacific herring	1.7	12	13.9
Atlantic herring	1.6	18	9.0
Lake trout	1.6	17	9.7
European anchovy	1.4	29	4.8
Atlantic salmon	1.2	22	5.4
Pink salmon	1.0	29	3.4
Striped bass	0.8	35	2.3
Pacific oyster	0.6	26	2.3
Blue mussels	0.5	22	2.2
Tuna	0.5	20	2.5
Rainbow trout	0.5	15	3.4
Pacific halibut	0.4	17	2.3
Atlantic cod	0.3	43	0.7
Alaska King crab	0.3	38	0.8
Dungeness crab	0.3	30	1.0
Shrimp	0.3	27	1.1
Catfish	0.3	7	4.3
Haddock	0.2	29	0.7
Scallops	0.2	25	0.8
Northern lobster	0.2	22	0.9
Flounder	0.2	20	1.0
Red snapper	0.2	17	1.2
Sole	0.1	8	1.2

"This could be due to several reasons," Terry says. "What is true in rodents, for example, or in a 'test tube' may not be true in free-living humans." Or perhaps you have to get a lot of omega-3s, but the studies couldn't examine levels that high. It is also possible that we lack the ability to accurately measure intakes of omega-3 fatty acids, Terry says.

But what if you cut way back on omega-6s and increased omega-3s? Only a little research has examined whether this tactic can help fight cancer — but that research seems to show promise. However, scientists need to study this more thoroughly to find out what works and what doesn't.

Become a fish expert

While researchers keep hunting for answers, you can work to win the battle between omega-3s and omega-6s. Every week, eat at least two servings of omega-3-packed fish, like salmon, herring, or canned light tuna.

The latest buzz on fish oil

Studies by two consumer organizations show that most fish oil supplements contain the EPA and DHA amounts claimed on the label and are free of contaminants. But talk with your doctor before you start taking them. These supplements may not be safe for folks with some health conditions or those who take certain medications or herbs.

For example, fish oil capsules might thin your blood too much if you take them with blood thinners, like Coumadin (warfarin), or NSAIDs, like ibuprofen and aspirin.

Very high doses of omega-3s can also increase bleeding time and may suppress the immune system. The FDA recommends you get no more than 2 grams of fish oil per day from supplements.

Omega-3s in fish may have other benefits to offer, too. In fact, one review of omega-3 research on cancer suggests following the American Heart Association recommendations for fish and fish oil supplements. Read *Omega-3 fatty acids for heart disease* (see below) to learn more about these recommendations and to net good advice on consuming fish and fish oil supplements safely.

But don't forget to take aim at the omega-6s that swarm into your diet. And eat less red meat, too. It's high in omega-6s and saturated fats.

According to the American Cancer Society, a high-fat diet increases your risk of colon, rectum, prostate, and endometrium (uterine lining) cancers.

> Albacore tuna tends to have a greater concentration of mercury than canned light tuna," says Sharon Alger-Mayer, physician-nutrition specialist and associate professor of medicine at Albany Medical College in New York. That's why light canned tuna is safer to eat.

Omega-3 fatty acids for heart disease ★★☆

Eat fish to tame heart trouble

Getting enough omega-3 fatty acids could help save your life. Find out how — and discover the little-known powers of these nutritious and heart-healthy fats.

How it works

Your body can't make omega-3 fatty acids, but you can get them from foods. Delicious cold water fish bring you two omega-3s — eicosapentaenoic acid (EPA) and docosahexaenoic acid (DHA). Meanwhile, landlubber foods like flaxseed and walnuts provide alpha-linolenic acid (ALA).

Scientists think omega-3s may work with your body to produce substances that stop potential heart attack triggers. These natural chemicals may help keep blood vessel walls flexible and prevent blood clots and inflammation in your arteries.

Best of all, these omega-3s may help prevent "sudden death" — death during the first hour after a heart attack. The American Heart Association (AHA) reports that 340,000 sudden deaths occur due to heart disease every year. Arrhythmia, an abnormal heartbeat rate, may cause most of these deaths. But EPA and DHA get into the heart's cells and help stabilize heart rate, explains Penny Kris-Etherton, Ph.D., distinguished professor of nutrition at Pennsylvania State University. And that may be enough to prevent the arrhythmia that leads to sudden death.

Hook a heart helper

In a recent American Heart Association review, Kris-Etherton and her colleagues examined the research on omega-3s. They concluded these fats can help reduce your risk of developing

Get the scoop on ALA

"The evidence for ALA clearly is not as strong as it is for EPA and DHA," says University of Pennsylvania Distinguished Professor of Nutrition Penny Kris-Etherton. "But there still is some evidence."

In a review of ALA's effectiveness against heart disease, scientists concluded that it may help prevent arrhythmias. Some research also suggests that very high intakes of ALA might possibly be linked to prostate cancer risk. But more research is needed to determine whether ALA truly raises prostate cancer odds and exactly how it might be used against heart disease.

New omega-3 claim for food labels

Getting more omega-3 fatty acids just got easier. Now you can check the labels of food products to find heart-healthy EPA and DHA fatty acids. Look for the following claim newly approved by the FDA — "Supportive but not conclusive research shows that consumption of EPA and DHA omega-3 fatty acids may reduce the risk of coronary heart disease."

If you see this claim on the package, check the nutrition information on the label or nearby signs or brochures to find out how much omega-3 fatty acids the product contains.

heart disease. Omega-3s can even help if you already have heart disease.

Several large studies have noted what happened when people with heart disease got enough omega-3s. Not only were there fewer deaths from heart disease, but also fewer deaths from other causes too, says Dr. Maggie Covington, a clinical assistant professor of family medicine at the University of Maryland with an integrative medicine practice in Bethesda, Maryland. While that doesn't mean omega-3s make you live forever, they may help you hang on to better health.

Fish oil tips and traps

The AHA recommends you eat a wide variety of fish high in omega-3s at least twice a week. Include other foods and oils rich in these fatty acids as well.

If you have documented heart disease, the AHA recommends as much as 1 gram of combined EPA and DHA daily. Get all you can from food, but the AHA suggests you ask your doctor about getting the rest from fish oil supplements. Yet, be a wise consumer of fish — or fish oil supplements — and know their risks and benefits.

"Be aware of the possible contaminants now in fish — particularly farm-raised," says Covington. Fish have become the main food sources of contaminants like mercury and polychlorinated biphenyls (PCBs). Most people don't eat enough fish to be in serious danger of mercury poisoning, but this metal can cause brain damage and interfere with the development of unborn and young children. The Food and Drug Administration (FDA) and the Environmental Protection Agency (EPA) recommend the following for children under 5 and women who may be pregnant or nursing.

- Don't eat high-mercury fish such as shark, swordfish, king mackerel, or tilefish.

- Eat up to 12 ounces (two meals) a week of a variety of low-mercury fish and shellfish.

- Check local advisories about the safety of fish caught in local lakes, rivers, and coastal waters. Otherwise, eat no more than 6 ounces of fish caught from local waters, and eat no other fish that week.

A new study suggests farmed salmon may contain more PCBs and other pollutants than wild salmon. Stay tuned to see if the FDA, EPA, and AHA update their recommendations in response to this study.

The AHA says the benefits of eating fish twice a week outweigh the risks for older men and post-menopausal women.

Oddly enough, fish oil supplements may be cleaner than fish. "There are a couple of studies that have been done that show that they are pure — they don't have environmental contaminants," Kris-Etherton says. And studies by two consumer organizations show that nearly all products contain the amount of EPA and DHA claimed on the label.

On the other hand, fish supplements can have side effects like gas, burping, and fishy aftertaste. "Usually that can be alleviated by starting at lower doses and working your way up," says Covington. But fish oil supplements may thin your blood, so talk to your doctor before taking them with other medications — particularly blood thinners such as Coumadin (Warfarin) and NSAIDs.

Omega-3 fatty acids for rheumatoid arthritis

Take the edge off tender joints

Imagine cutting back on the anti-inflammatory drugs you take for rheumatoid arthritis — or having fewer tender joints or less morning stiffness. Special oils found in delicious fish might make this possible in just a few months.

How it works

Rheumatoid arthritis (RA) inflames your joints, causing tenderness. Fortunately, you might help your body resist inflammation with the omega-3 fatty acids found in fish and other foods.

"The omega-3 fats are involved in the production of many chemicals in the body that control inflammation," says Sharon Alger-Mayer, physician-nutrition specialist and associate professor of medicine at Albany Medical College in New York. "Chemicals that are produced through the omega-3 fats tend to be much less inflammatory than chemicals that are produced by the omega-6 fatty acids."

Unfortunately, modern diets are loaded with omega-6. It's in corn oil, safflower oil, eggs, meat, milk, and fried or processed foods. In fact, you could be getting up to 25 times more omega-6 than omega-3.

You can get two omega-3s from fish — eicosapentaenoic acid (EPA) and docosahexaenoic acid (DHA). Landlubber foods like flaxseed and walnuts contain another omega-3 oil — alpha-linolenic acid or ALA. But ALA may pack less punch. "It probably is going to require more of that type of oil to get the same benefit that you would in a fish oil supplement," Alger-Mayer says.

Eggstasy, EggsPlus, Eggland's Best, or Choice Eggs are all special brands of egg that give you a helping of omega-3s — but they're expensive and probably won't give you as much omega-3s as fish.

Ease the pain

According to a review by the Agency for Healthcare Research and Quality, six out of seven studies suggested that fish oils might reduce the need for anti-inflammatory drugs. But the report found no evidence that fish oils can cure or lessen RA— or even affect most symptoms.

However, other reviews suggest omega-3s might help reduce the number of tender joints from RA and may reduce morning stiffness. But patience is key. You'll probably need to get 3 grams of fish oil per day for 12 weeks before you can expect results. "The process takes time," says Alger-Mayer. These new, less-inflammatory chemicals need to be incorporated into our tissues."

Serve up seafood with savvy

Make foods your first source of omega-3s. "Food matters. Food is medicine — and the kind of choices we make have a profound effect on our health," says Alger-Mayer.

The American Heart Association and the Arthritis Foundation both recommend eating fish twice a week. But don't just eat more fish. Saturated fats and omega-6 fats encourage inflammation, so cut back. Replace vegetable oils — like corn, safflower, soybean, and cottonseed — with olive or canola oils when you cook. In fact, olive oil may give you an extra boost in your fight against inflammation.

Next, cut back on processed and fast foods. "If you're going to McDonald's during the day, having Big Macs twice a day, taking 1,000 milligrams of fish oil at the end of the day is probably not going to cut it for you," Alger-Mayer says.

"There's been some very interesting studies in the psychiatric literature of the benefit of the omega-3s in helping with certain types of depression," says Sharon Alger-Mayer physician-nutrition specialist and Albany Medical College professor. "So individuals who are taking these supplements may get some added benefit."

Finally, replace meats with fish occasionally, but choose fish carefully. "Fish high up on the food chain — like shark, swordfish, king mackerel, and tilefish — have been shown to contain particularly high levels of mercury, and those are actually not recommended in pregnant women, nursing women, or young children," says Alger-Mayer.

Stick with low-mercury fish, like catfish, cod, salmon, tilapia, haddock, herring, scallops, anchovies, sardines, and whitefish. To learn more about choosing fish and fish oil supplements wisely, see *Omega-3 fatty acids for heart disease* on page 241.

Once you're getting as much omega-3 from food as you safely can, consider whether you need fish oil supplements. The FDA recommends no more than 3 grams of omega-3s per day — with no more than 2 grams from supplements.

Talk with your doctor before taking fish oil supplements. "You can take too much," says Alger-Mayer. "Very, very high doses of the omega-3s can have some detrimental effects. They can increase bleeding time. They have an effect on our platelets, and they can also cause a suppression of the immune system when taken in very high doses."

Eat 'miracle meals' to fend off disease

Sometimes the best natural remedies can be found right in your own kitchen! Many people have found that by adding just the right delicious foods to their diets, they are able to reduce or even stop taking prescription drugs for good.

Why pop prescription pills when there's a wonder food that can fight rheumatoid arthritis, heart disease, type 2 diabetes, stomach disorders, mental problems, and even protect against certain cancers. Fish — with their omega-3 fatty acids — might be the right food for your health concerns.

For example, omega-3s help process insulin. Without them, you risk developing insulin resistance — often a first step toward diabetes and high blood sugar. For more examples, read *Omega-3 fatty acids for rheumatoid arthritis* (see page 245), *Omega-3 fatty acids for cancer* (see page 237), and *Omega-3 fatty acids for heart disease* (see page 241).

To add omega-3s, replace meat with fish twice a week and substitute nuts or seeds for snacks high in saturated fat. If this sheers saturated fat from your diet, it may also slice cholesterol, lower high blood pressure, help prevent cancer, and ease the "sour stomach" of acid indigestion. And that could lead to a long life — free from cancer, disease, and arthritis pain.

Ornish program for heart disease ★★☆

Cleanse your arteries

Can it really be done? Dr. Dean Ornish testified to the U.S. Senate that his program had shown some reversal of coronary artery plaque buildup after one year — and even more after five years.

"The program has proven to improve blood flow to the heart by promoting plaque regression," says Jennifer Grana, a registered dietician with Highmark, Inc., who helps oversee the Ornish program in Pennsylvania hospitals. In participants in the Ornish program, this is measured by decreased chest pain and improvement in stress tests, she says.

Find out if this highly effective, all-natural treatment can flush plaque and fatty buildup out of your arteries, too.

How it works

Blood clots, clogged arteries, constricted arteries, or artery spasms can limit blood flow to the heart and could trigger a heart attack. The Ornish program might help prevent these heart attack triggers.

Too much cholesterol in your blood encourages artery-clogging deposits to build up. Your "bad" LDL cholesterol level can skyrocket if your diet is high in saturated fat and cholesterol. Fortunately, your liver cells have LDL receptors that can bind and remove cholesterol, and "good" HDL cholesterol helps purge LDL, too. But they often can't work fast enough to beat the LDL overload from a poor diet. Under Ornish's program, you eat so little cholesterol and fat that your body might never have more LDL than it can eliminate.

But that's not all. Stress causes your body to release adrenaline and other hormones that increase your heart rate and raise your blood pressure, which can cause constrictions or spasms in your arteries. "There's a lot of research out there, too, that shows that hostility, isolation, and depression actually contribute to heart disease," says Grana. Both stress management and exercise help lower blood pressure, but exercise also helps promote weight loss and improve blood flow to your heart.

These guidelines summarize the Ornish program.

- no more than 10 percent of total calories from fat and only 5 milligrams of cholesterol per day

---

8 ways to tackle triglycerides

Triglycerides are fats that provide fuel for your body. However, studies have linked high triglyceride levels with heart disease. Here are eight things you can do to reduce triglycerides and lower your risk for heart disease.
- Maintain a healthy weight by balancing the calories you take in with the calories you burn.
- Exercise regularly.
- Limit sweets and eat more whole grains.
- Eat high-fiber foods, like dried beans, vegetables, and fruits.
- Reduce saturated fat, found mainly in meat and dairy products, in your diet to less than 35 percent of your daily calories. The American Heart Association warns that cutting total fat to less than 15 percent of daily calories may boost triglycerides.
- Eat two 6-ounce servings of fatty fish, like salmon, sardines, mackerel, and tuna, weekly and ask your doctor about fish oil supplements.
- Quit smoking.
- If you drink, stay at or below the recommended daily limit of two drinks — containing one-half ounce of pure alcohol — if you're a male and one drink if you're female.

- plenty of fiber and plant foods, like fruits, vegetables, grains, and legumes

- little alcohol and no caffeine

- no oils or animal products except nonfat milk, yogurt, and egg whites

- minimal salt and sugar

- moderate daily aerobic exercise

- stress management training

- group support meetings

- no smoking

Heal your heart

Is it possible to reverse heart disease naturally in 365 days or less? Ornish's research suggests the answer might be yes. In eight out of every 10 patients studied, the arteries that had been clogged were cleaner, according to one research project.

In addition, an early test of the Ornish program found that in only 24 days participants experienced these amazing results.

- reduced chest pain by 91 percent

- improved ability to exercise

- reduced cholesterol levels by 21 percent

- lessened anxiety, fear, and depression

But there's more good news about this drug-free remedy. In three research studies, Ornish had to decrease or discontinue blood pressure medications for most participants. Their diet and lifestyle changes had brought down their blood pressure naturally. If you or someone you know has high blood pressure, this drug-free remedy could be worth checking out.

Ornish's latest research included 440 participants across the country. As with previous studies, the participants lowered LDL cholesterol, weight, and blood pressure and increased their ability to exercise. Their triglyceride levels didn't change, and their HDL cholesterol dropped but returned to starting levels by the study's end.

Most eating programs supported by the American Heart Association (AHA) recommend a total fat intake of no more than 30 percent of total calories. But AHA does not recommend diets with less than 15 percent of fat from calories because short-term studies suggest these diets can raise triglycerides and reduce HDL cholesterol. No long-term studies have examined the safety and effectiveness of these very-low-fat diets.

But Ornish's exciting research results are from people who didn't just use the diet. "The stress management, exercise, and group support are certainly extremely effective in the fight against heart disease and the goal to reverse it," says Grana.

Get expert advice

Talk with your doctor before you try the Ornish program. It isn't right for everyone. The Ornish diet is pretty strict, so plan ahead. You might have a hard time cutting meat and fats, including olive oil, and avoiding sugar and salt.

Getting enough fresh, unprocessed foods will be a challenge in today's on-the-go society. Watch your nutrient intake to make sure you don't become deficient in calcium or vitamins E, B12, and D. And eat a variety of vegetarian protein sources — like rice with beans — to meet your body's amino acid requirements. Finally, allow several hours for exercise and stress management every week.

To find out more, call 800-879-2217 if you're in West Virginia or Pennsylvania — or 800-775-7674 if you live in other states.

Prayer for high blood pressure ★ ★ ★

Humble the 'silent killer'

More people use prayer than any other complementary medicine — more than meditation, chiropractic, yoga, herbs, or dietary supplements. What's more, research is proving that prayer has the power to help control even the silent killer — high blood pressure.

How it works

High blood pressure, also known as hypertension, affects one in three American adults. Many people don't know they have it because it usually doesn't cause any symptoms. The only way to know for sure if your blood pressure is high is to have it checked regularly.

The causes aren't clear, but health experts think stress is a contributing factor. If you've ever been stressed, chances are you've taken a brisk walk or relaxed in a hot tub to unwind. Activities like these not only relieve your stress, they relax your blood vessels and lower your blood pressure. Strange as it may seem, prayer can do the same thing.

Change the way you breathe

Never underestimate the power of prayer. Medical research confirms its healing power. A study reported in a British medical journal says praying calms your heart and lowers your blood pressure by changing the way you breathe.

Normally, you take about 14 breaths a minute. This drops to eight when you're carrying on normal conversation. But studies show your breathing rate can drop to six when you pray. Researchers say this slower respiration rate has a positive effect on your heart and lungs.

Reciting repetitive prayers, like the Rosary, can stabilize your breathing and harmonize your heart's rhythms.

Another study of 3,963 people age 65 and older found that those who participated in religious activities, like prayer, were 40 percent less likely to have high blood pressure than people who didn't. The research also shows that prayerful people are inclined to be more positive and hopeful, which can result in a slower heart rate, improved breathing, and lower blood pressure.

Not surprisingly, those who hold on to anger and are reluctant to forgive have higher blood pressure. The burden they bear, borne by the heart and arteries over a period of years, can eventually lead to heart disease. Pray for the wisdom and courage to

Spice up your life without salt

Food	Experiment with new flavors
Fish	basil, curry powder, dill, garlic, lemon juice, dry mustard, nutmeg, paprika, parsley, sage, or turmeric
Chicken	curry powder, dill, ginger, dry mustard, nutmeg, or rosemary
Lean meat	allspice, bay leaves, caraway seeds, chives, curry powder, garlic, lemon juice, dry mustard, onion, paprika, parsley, sage, thyme, or turmeric
Soups	basil, bay leaves, caraway seeds, chives, dill, garlic, onions, paprika, parsley, or thyme
Stews	allspice, basil, bay leaves, caraway seeds, or sage
Sauces	basil, chives, cider vinegar, dry mustard, paprika, parsley, rosemary, thyme, or turmeric
Vegetables	chives, cider vinegar, garlic, lemon juice, onion, paprika, or parsley

Courtesy of the American Heart Association

forgive past grievances. Releasing anger and resentment can help you heal.

Complement your traditional treatments

If you have high blood pressure, follow your doctor's orders to keep it under control. Prayer doesn't replace standard medical treatments, like diet, exercise, and medication — but it could help them work better.

There may be times when you want to pray but can't find the words. There are many helpful books and Web sites to help you heal yourself with prayer. The Bible's book of Psalms is a good place to start.

Prescription drugs for hair loss ★★★

2 ways to reverse baldness

You're clearly losing the battle against baldness. Time to call in the heavy artillery. The biggest success in reversing hair loss has come from powerhouse prescription drugs like finasteride and minoxidil, the only two hair loss remedies approved by the FDA. Both can help your hair survive to fight another day.

How it works

Finasteride, better known as Propecia, seems to work by counteracting the process that converts testosterone into the hormone known as dihydrotestosterone (DHT).

If you have a family history of baldness, it's especially important to prevent the formation of DHT because having too much in your scalp tissue will definitely result in hair loss. DHT destroys the blood supply to your hair, shrinking the hair follicles to the point where hair growth is no longer possible.

Scientists have dubbed this process "progressive miniaturization." Finasteride seems to help by blocking the enzyme 5-alpha-reductase, which sets the whole process in motion.

Because the affected hair follicles become dormant, not dead, they can be stimulated to resume growth. This may be where the drug minoxidil finds success.

Sold under the brand name Rogaine, minoxidil is a popular topical remedy, although it's not clear how it promotes hair regrowth. It's thought to increase hair density either by stimulating the growth stage of hair development or making it last longer.

Minoxidil also seems to increase the thickness of the hair strands. The result is that it may reverse the miniaturization process, slow the progression of hair loss, or both.

Studies show hair grows

Both minoxidil and finasteride have been extensively tested — and, for the most part, passed with flying colors.

- Several studies have determined that 2-percent minoxidil stimulates hair growth and prevents further hair loss in both men and women.

- A recent study comparing 2-percent minoxidil and 5-percent minoxidil showed the stronger formula works even better and quicker. After 48 weeks, men using the 5-percent solution saw 45-percent more hair regrowth.

- A similar study showed less-impressive results for women. While the 5-percent solution beat the placebo, it was not markedly better than the 2-percent solution. It also caused more side effects.

- Men ages 18 to 41 who take finasteride for one year consistently boost their scalp coverage and hair counts compared to placebo.

- After two years of daily finasteride treatment, two-thirds of men improve hair regrowth, one-third show no change, and about 1 percent have less hair. Men under 60 get better results.

- Finasteride does not fare as well with women. It actually increased hair loss in one study and had no effect in another.

Beware of cost, side effects

Now you can buy Rogaine or generic minoxidil without a prescription in the United States. Men have the option of the standard 2-percent or 5-percent extra-strength version. The stronger solution has not yet been approved for women.

To use, follow the dosage directions on the label. Just make sure your hair and scalp are dry. If you are under age 18 or over age 65, ask your doctor for the proper dosage.

Possible side effects include itching, scalp irritation, and facial hair growth in women.

Finasteride requires a prescription, so you'll need to talk with your doctor and follow his directions. Possible side effects include decreased sex drive and impotence. Finasteride can also cause birth defects in male fetuses. That's why it's not approved for women.

Both drugs come with a hefty pricetag. It will cost about $10 to $20 a month for minoxidil and $30 to $60 a month for finasteride.

Once you start treatment with either drug, you can't stop — unless you're ready to surrender the baldness battle. Hair loss begins again shortly after you stop treatment.

Probiotics for IBD

Bacteria battle inflammation

You probably think of bacteria as the enemy. You wash your hands with anti-bacterial soap, scrub your house with anti-bacterial cleaning products, and make sure to handle and cook food safely to avoid bacteria.

But bacteria aren't always bad. In fact, some can be quite good. These good bacteria, called probiotics, may help treat inflammatory bowel disease (IBD), which includes both ulcerative colitis and Crohn's disease.

Ulcerative colitis involves inflammation of the colon and rectum, while Crohn's disease can affect your entire intestinal tract, from mouth to rectum. Symptoms include rectal pain and cramping, bloody diarrhea, stomach pain, nausea, appetite loss, weight loss, and fever.

Far from being your enemy, probiotics may be valuable allies in your fight against these serious conditions.

How it works

Your gastrointestinal tract contains hundreds of different species of harmless bacteria. If you get sick or take antibiotics, you lower the numbers of these beneficial bacteria in your system. This disturbance of the normal balance can lead to diarrhea and other intestinal problems.

Certain bacteria used to ferment dairy products such as yogurt are powerful disease fighters with anti-inflammatory properties. These microorganisms are called "probiotics" because they exert health benefits over and above basic nutrition. They help restore the balance of good bacteria to your gut by flooding your small intestine and crowding out the harmful bacteria.

Scientists think they also may have other benefits that work against the bad bacteria and help stimulate your body's immune system to fight them off.

Keep symptoms at bay

The strongest evidence for probiotics comes from a special strain of *E. coli* and a product called VSL#3. Normally you want to avoid *E. coli*, which can cause serious infection. But one particular strain — *Escherichia coli (E. coli)* Nissle 1917, sold under the brand name Mutaflor — helps maintain remission in IBD.

- It was twice as effective as a placebo in a study of people with Crohn's disease. Only one-third of those taking Mutaflor had a relapse, compared to two-thirds of those taking the placebo.

- Mutaflor was as safe and effective as the drug mesalamine, the standard IBD treatment, in a recent study of people with ulcerative colitis.

VSL#3, which includes four strains of *Lactobacillus*, three strains of *Bifidobacterium*, and one strain of *Streptococci*, provides 450 billion live bacteria in each 6-gram dose. It also provides relief for IBD.

- In a study of 20 people with ulcerative colitis in remission, 15 remained in remission for one year while taking 3 grams of VSL#3 twice daily.

- People with Crohn's disease taking VSL#3 for one year had only a 20-percent risk of relapse compared to a 30-percent risk for those taking mesalamine.

- Studies show VSL#3 helps with pouchitis. This is a common complication of a surgical procedure to remove diseased large intestines in people with severe ulcerative colitis. Half of those who undergo this surgery experience inflammation of the pouch inserted to connect the small intestine and anus.

---

5 ways to ease IBD

Inflammatory bowel disease is a serious condition calling for real medical intervention, so you should talk to your doctor about medicine and a full treatment plan. However, with his approval, you can make some diet and lifestyle changes that may minimize your symptoms.

- High-fiber foods will probably give you cramps, diarrhea, and grumpy intestines, since your colon is already narrowed and inflamed. Stay away from beans, corn, raisins, raw vegetables, whole grains, and raw fruits.
- Avoid high-fat foods that can cause cramping and diarrhea.
- Certain hot or spicy foods may aggravate your digestive system. Track what you eat to identify your triggers.
- Many people with IBD are lactose intolerant — meaning they don't have enough of a specific enzyme that breaks down dairy products. These foods will probably make you miserable.
- Try eating five, or even six, small meals each day, instead of three large ones.

Not all probiotic studies are positive, though. Much more research is needed before probiotics become standard treatment for IBD.

Become a billionaire

Aim high. Experts say you need 1 billion to 10 billion good bacteria per day. Luckily, that's easy to do. One cup of yogurt should do the trick. Look for products with live active cultures. Another way to get your probiotics is by drinking them. Actimel, a fermented milk drink popular in Europe, is now available in the U.S. as DanActive.

You can also buy probiotic supplements in drug stores and supermarkets without a prescription. Read the label to see which bacteria you're getting. Keep in mind the label might not read "probiotics," but it should say it contains bacteria or promotes healthy digestion. Don't be confused by the numbers on the label. One billion may be written as 10^9 or 1×10^9.

Probiotic supplements are not regulated by the FDA, so you can't really be sure what you're getting. In a recent test, one-third of probiotic products contained less than 1 percent of the expected 1 billion bacteria. Those that listed the expected amount of bacteria at the time of use, as opposed to time of manufacture, fared better.

Pay attention to the label's expiration date. You want to make sure the bacteria are still alive. Store products in the refrigerator to extend their shelf life.

Prolotherapy for chronic pain

Strengthen weak ligaments

You might rid yourself of chronic pain with a revolutionary therapy. If you've tried everything else with no success, this simple treatment could be your key to freedom from constant pain.

How it works

"Weakened ligaments and tendons are believed to be a common cause of chronic joint pain," says Dr. Michael Yelland, senior lecturer in general practice, University of Queensland, Australia, and a practitioner of musculoskeletal medicine.

If either one is stretched because of trauma, it's not able to snap back into shape. This leaves you with a weakened, loose joint. "Prolotherapy injections aim to strengthen these weak ligaments by restarting your healing process," Yelland says.

> Prolotherapy uses the process of inflammation to help repair ligaments and tendons. So don't use NSAIDs, like ibuprofen or aspirin, after having prolotherapy. They may provide you with short-term pain relief, but they'll inhibit your body's repair work.

The irritant injected into the tissue causes mild inflammation in your ligament. "The inflammation stimulates the body to strengthen these weakened ligaments with strong fibers called collagen," says Yelland. New collagen shrinks as it matures. The shrinking collagen tightens the ligament, which results in stronger, thicker ligaments and tendons.

Lasting pain relief

Yelland and his colleagues recently completed a two-year prolotherapy study in Brisbane, Australia, involving 110 volunteers. They looked at how helpful the treatments were in relieving chronic low back pain.

In the study, the researchers used a solution of 20 percent glucose (a sugar) and .2 percent lignocaine (a painkiller) or a placebo of saline (salt water). Treatments included injections every two weeks for four to six months.

The participants were also randomly assigned to perform bending exercises or continue their normal activities.

At 12 months, there were no major differences between the glucose group and the saline group, regardless of physical activity.

- Of the people who experienced a 50-percent reduction in pain, 46 percent received the glucose solution and 36 percent received the saline.

- 75 percent of the participants said they had less pain than when they started the treatment.

- 20 percent of the people said they no longer had low-back pain.

Since both solutions worked, Yelland and his colleagues are not sure if the needle or the solution acted as the irritant. Either way, the ligament became inflamed, which started the healing process.

Things you need to know

Besides back pain, prolotherapy has been used to relieve pain caused by migraines, fibromyalgia, and osteoarthritis.

Prolotherapists claim this simple, drug-free, nonsurgical procedure can also relieve neck pain, dizziness, nausea, blurred vision, and tinnitus.

Prolotherapy should be part of a whole treatment program. Exercise, massage, and taking vitamin and mineral supplements are also encouraged during and after treatments, says Yelland.

Most people need four to six prolotherapy sessions. Yet, some people feel pain relief after the first treatment. For maximum

---

Smile to stop the pain

Doctors agree that your state of mind affects your ability to handle chronic pain. An upbeat attitude and an active lifestyle work wonders. Here are a few more ways to help reduce your chronic pain.

- Try the holistic approach with yoga. It's already being touted as a way to help those with chronic problems. A recent study concluded that a modified yoga-based program may benefit individuals with chronic low back pain.
- Laugh. Besides boosting your immune system, relieving stress, and chasing away anger, laughter can help you keep a positive attitude through difficult times.
- Write about it. The pen is mightier than the sword — and it may help slay pain. Research suggests that writing about stressful events in your life may help improve your condition.

benefit, experts recommend spreading your sessions several weeks apart.

Currently, Medicare does not cover the cost of prolotherapy. Some insurance companies may reimburse you after you've gone through the treatments, but some will not. Check with your insurance company before starting the therapy.

The cost of prolotherapy can vary. One session of multiple injections costs around $200 — add another $40 for additional areas.

Prolotherapy is not a cure-all for every kind of pain. That's why it is essential to get an accurate diagnosis from your doctor, and, if you decide to try it, only receive treatment from a trained prolotherapist.

To locate a prolotherapist, contact the American Association of Orthopaedic Medicine at 800-992-2063, or find one online at *www.aaomed.org* or *www.getprolo.com*.

Psyllium for diabetes

⭐⭐⭐

Fabulous fiber controls blood sugar

You've probably heard of using psyllium to stay regular. But this soluble fiber found in Metamucil and other bulk laxatives also helps regulate your blood sugar and cholesterol levels. With that kind of one-two punch, psyllium can help knock out diabetes.

How it works

Slow and steady wins the race. That's the secret of psyllium's success. Technically an herb derived from the husk of psyllium seed, psyllium forms a gel that slows the digestion of food as it moves through your system. Because it takes longer to break down carbohydrates and absorb glucose into your bloodstream, insulin has more time to convert that glucose into energy.

Psyllium likely lowers cholesterol by decreasing the absorption of fat and cholesterol, increasing bile acid, and inhibiting production of cholesterol by the liver.

Cholesterol plummets, blood sugar drops

Studies of psyllium have yielded some amazing results. Here are just a few examples.

- Controlling cholesterol a major concern? Here's good news. This natural substance has been shown to lower LDL cholesterol levels by up to 13 percent — and it lowers blood sugar levels by almost 20 percent. These eye-popping numbers come from a study by the Veterans Affairs Medical Center at the University of Kentucky in which 34 diabetic men took 10.2 grams of psyllium a day for eight weeks.

- A Spanish study of 12 men and eight women with diabetes reported encouraging results as well. After taking 14 grams of psyllium a day for six weeks, they saw their glucose absorption decrease by 12 percent. However, results varied greatly between individuals. Their total cholesterol (7.7 percent) and LDL cholesterol (9.2 percent) also dropped significantly.

- Dozens of clinical trials have shown psyllium lowers total and LDL cholesterol. In fact, the mountain of evidence convinced the FDA to approve the following health claim: "Diets low in saturated fat and cholesterol that include soluble fiber from psyllium seed husk may reduce the risk of heart disease."

Then again, not all studies are positive. Adding 1.7 grams of psyllium to a serving of pasta did not have any effect on insulin or glucose in an English study.

Take charge of diabetes

You may have to take medication to help control your blood sugar levels, but that won't be enough. You must become committed to smart health choices.

- Get down to and maintain a healthy weight.
- Exercise regularly.
- Eat plenty of fiber.
- Don't skip meals or snacks.
- Take special care of your feet. Report problems to your doctor.
- Stop smoking.
- Limit alcohol.
- Avoid high-glycemic foods, such as candy and refined grains.

---

3 teaspoons a day does the trick

It's not hard to get psyllium into your diet. Besides Metamucil and bulk laxatives, you can also find psyllium as a food additive in breakfast cereals, such as Kellogg's Bran Buds.

That doesn't mean you should go silly for psyllium. Just one teaspoon, or about 5 grams, with water three times a day before meals can help reduce blood cholesterol levels and control blood sugar levels in diabetics. Follow the directions, and talk to your doctor before supplementing your diet with psyllium.

Psyllium has no serious side effects. Just make sure to drink plenty of water. As with any fiber, don't add too much of it to your diet too quickly. Otherwise, you might experience bloating or diarrhea.

SAMe for osteoarthritis pain

★★☆

Relief for stiff, achy joints

SAMe, discovered in Italy in 1952, has been used in Europe for decades and is finally gaining popularity in the United States. This naturally occurring biochemical can increase your mobility, ease your joint pain, and reduce inflammation. And best of all, you don't need a prescription for it.

How it works

Every cell of your body contains SAMe, or S-adenosyl-methionine. What's more, your body makes this amazing chemical. It's manufactured from methionine, an amino acid found in protein-rich foods, like meat, fish, dry beans, nuts, and dairy products.

Your joint's cartilage cells use SAMe to produce a gel-like substance that acts like a shock absorber. A deficiency of SAMe in your joints can affect this shock-absorbing ability, worsening your osteoarthritis. That's why SAMe supplements are becoming a popular treatment for osteoarthritis.

As effective as NSAIDs

In recent years, SAMe was best known for improving mood and feelings of well-being in people suffering with depression. And here's why — SAMe is involved in the production of serotonin, dopamine, and norepinephrine, neurotransmitters that play a role in depression.

While treating people with depression, researchers discovered SAMe also relieved the pain and stiffness of osteoarthritis.

In a recent meta-analysis, researchers examined the results of SAMe supplements when compared to a placebo or NSAIDs (non-steroidal anti-inflammatory drugs), like aspirin and ibuprofen.

In these studies, the SAMe dosage ranged from 600 to 1,200 milligrams (mg) for the 1,442 study participants. Although the average length of the studies was short — about 30 days — researchers concluded that SAMe increased mobility and worked as well as NSAIDs in relieving pain.

The study participants taking SAMe also reported fewer serious side effects, like stomach and intestinal bleeding, as those taking NSAIDs.

You'll probably be hearing more about SAMe in the future. Scientists think it might even repair damaged cartilage, but studies have not proven this yet.

What to watch out for

If you're looking for a quick fix, you better look elsewhere. SAMe doesn't work quickly. Improvements in symptoms can take a few days to five weeks.

Some health professionals recommend starting with 200 mg to 400 mg of SAMe a day, then increasing the dosage to 200 mg two to fours times a day.

Why agonize over surgery when you can heal back pain with this everyday beverage. Water acts as a cushion for all the joints of your body, including the disks of your spine. If your back hurts, try this old-fashioned remedy first.

SAMe supplements are expensive, and many experts are concerned about quality. Yet, Consumer Lab, an independent testing facility, recently tested 11 brands and only one did not have the label's stated amount.

It's always a good idea to talk with your doctor before using any supplement, including SAMe. Here are a few other things to keep in mind:

- To prevent nausea and upset stomach when taking SAMe, use enteric-coated products. They are formulated to break down in your intestines instead of your stomach.

- Don't take more than the recommended amount. High doses can cause gas, nausea, vomiting, diarrhea, and headache.

- Make sure you are getting enough vitamin B12, B6, and folate. These B-vitamins work closely with SAMe. Fortified breakfast cereals, tuna, whole-wheat bread, baked potatoes, and mushrooms are good sources.

- Follow your doctor's advice if you are taking an antidepressant, like MAO inhibitors, SSRIs, or tricyclics.

- Think twice about using SAMe if you have Parkinson's disease and are taking Levodopa. While SAMe can relieve Levodopa's side effects, it might also reduce its effectiveness.

- Don't use SAMe if you have bipolar disorder, or manic depression, because it could trigger a manic phase.

Saw palmetto for BPH

★★★

Nutritious berry helps prostate

Men with benign prostatic hyperplasia (BPH) are finding that saw palmetto — a food staple for centuries — may work just as well as the modern medicines and surgical techniques available today.

A small palm tree native to Florida and the West Indies, saw palmetto is also known as the dwarf palm. Early inhabitants of South Florida based their diet around saw palmetto's nutritious berries. Europeans apparently didn't like them as well, though.

A group of shipwrecked Quakers wrote in the late 1700s that they tasted like "rotten cheese steeped in tobacco juice."

The Seminole Indians used saw palmetto for an aphrodisiac, and an 1892 report stated it "exerts a great influence over the organs of reproduction." By the late 1920s, doctors began to recognize saw palmetto's positive effect on the bladder, prostate, and urethra, and specifically recommended it for enlarged prostate cases.

How it works

Symptoms of BPH affect half of all men by the time they're 75. It causes urinary flow problems because the prostate gland

Manage BPH naturally

Benign prostatic hyperplasia (BPH) can be a nuisance and it can lead to more serious problems. Talk to your doctor about medical intervention — surgery or drugs — and consider these natural treatments.

- Your prostate contains more zinc than any other part of your body and some believe this mineral could relieve symptoms of BPH. Talk to your doctor about getting more zinc from foods or supplements.
- Pumpkin seeds contain natural chemicals that interfere with prostate growth. Eat a handful every day to improve urinary problems.
- Research shows pygeum — from the African plum tree — is an effective remedy. Take 50 to 100 milligrams twice daily.
- An extract from the stinging nettle plant may reduce BPH symptoms without side effects. The recommended dose is 150 to 300 milligrams daily.
- Avoid medications that contain decongestants. They can make urinary symptoms worse.
- Limit caffeine and alcohol, especially late in the afternoon.

becomes enlarged and squeezes the urethra, the tube that carries urine out of the body. Saw palmetto supplements are mainly used to improve urinary flow and reduce the frequent and urgent need to urinate.

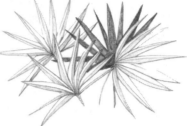

The oily compounds found in its berries give this herb its value as a medicine. It's believed that fatty acids in extracts of the berries block testosterone from causing the prostate to grow. Sterols in the saw palmetto berry also contribute to the positive effect, although their specific role is not clearly understood. By acting to keep the prostate at a more normal size, this herbal supplement helps relieve the problems associated with BPH.

A successful, natural remedy

In recent years, saw palmetto has been pushed aside as a BPH treatment by synthetic drugs that are more powerful, more popular, and more expensive. But a long history of use in Europe and several positive studies give solid support for its effectiveness.

It's also the only phytotherapeutic agent — plant-based healing substance — with solid evidence that it's effective against BPH.

A recent survey of 21 randomized studies examining more than 3,000 men with BPH found that men taking saw palmetto were 76 percent more likely to have improved urinary symptoms than those taking a placebo. It also said saw palmetto produced urinary symptom and peak urine flow results similar to the drug finasteride — with fewer side effects.

Finasteride is one of two equally effective drugs for BPH called 5-alpha-reductase inhibitors. Alpha-blockers also are used to treat both BPH and high blood pressure. Several small studies suggest saw palmetto may be as effective as alpha-blockers, too.

Buy it at the grocery store

Saw palmetto is a dietary supplement — not a drug — so no governmental or independent agency requires it to be tested for quality. Look for it at health food stores or in the health and beauty sections of drug stores, grocery stores, and discount stores. A month's supply will probably cost from $4 to $20, a fraction of the price of a prescription drug.

The normal dose is 320 milligrams per day of saw palmetto berry extract. It should contain 85 to 95 percent fatty acids and 0.2 to 0.4 percent sterols to be effective.

Be sure and let your doctor know you are taking saw palmetto, especially if you don't notice improvement within about six weeks. Prostate cancer has some of the same symptoms as BPH, and you need to be sure you're treating the right disease.

Shark cartilage for cancer

Beware of fishy remedy

A book called *Sharks Don't Get Cancer* generated quite a stir a few years ago by promoting shark cartilage as a miracle cure for cancer. Since sharks didn't get cancer, it said, their cartilage could help your body fight it off, too.

The problem is, no one knows for sure if shark cartilage has any effect at all on cancer. Claims of the healing power of both shark and cattle cartilage have gone along with the rising popularity of complementary and alternative medicines.

About the only thing creditable research says for sure is:

- it is possible for sharks to get cancer, and
- shark cartilage has no effect on advanced-stage cancer.

One researcher points out the world's shark population has suffered because the fish are being killed for their cartilage. He says, too, that cancer patients are missing out on legitimate treatment options by taking shark cartilage instead.

How it works

After researchers proved sharks do get cancer, other theories emerged as to why their cartilage may help battle this disease. Researchers point out that cancer cells rarely invade cartilage, possibly due to substances that inhibit the destruction of collagen. It's also possible cartilage's density coupled with fewer blood vessels make it less hospitable to cancer cell growth.

A more common theory is that a protein in the cartilage may help prevent angiogenesis — the growth of new blood vessels — that nourish tumors. Others think something within the cartilage stimulates the immune system to fight off tumor cells.

But much more research needs to be done to verify whether these potential anticancer components can truly help.

Studies offer no proof

The Chinese have used shark fin soup to cure many ailments for more than 100 years. And scientists in the U.S. have been interested in cattle cartilage for healing wounds for nearly 50 years. But whether these substances can help cure cancer is another matter.

The National Cancer Institute (NCI) reports more than a dozen studies of cow or shark cartilage since the 1970s. None of them have provided reliable evidence that either one works as a treatment for cancer.

Experts say that simply taking a small pill of crude extract won't pass those properties on to humans. They also point out that stomach acid destroys the protein that prevents blood vessel growth. Even if it survives the acid, the actual protein molecule is too big to get into your bloodstream, so it just passes on through your body.

The NCI's official position is that it cannot recommend cartilage, unless it is taken as part of a well-designed study. Several FDA-approved studies are underway as scientists try to isolate the particular properties of cartilage that show promise as cancer preventors.

A dietary supplement

Shark cartilage is not a drug. The Food and Drug Administration (FDA) classifies it as a dietary supplement and does not approve it for the treatment of cancer or anything else. No disease prevention claims are allowed, so there is no evidence it's effective. More than 40 different brand names are sold in the United States. Because they have no standard quality requirement, the exact makeup of each brand can be different.

If you choose to take this supplement, you may experience mild side effects such as digestive discomfort, weakness, low blood pressure, or hyperglycemia. A problem to watch out for, though,

---

Strengthen your cancer defense

There may be specific ways to battle specific cancers, but generally, here's how to give your body its best fighting chance against this deadly disease.

- Exercise regularly.
- Don't smoke.
- Avoid alcohol.
- Lower your fat intake.
- Increase fiber to 20 to 30 grams a day.
- Eat more fruits and vegetables.
- Balance the essential fatty acids in your body by eating more cold-water fish, flaxseed, and walnuts.

is hypercalcemia — too much calcium in the blood. Doctors have seen this in cancer patients who take large doses of vitamin D, calcium supplements, or calcium-rich shark cartilage.

Symptoms of hypercalcemia are fatigue, depression, mental confusion, nausea, vomiting, constipation, and increased urination. See your doctor immediately if you suspect this condition.

St. John's wort for depression

Herbal remedy fights the blues

St. John's wort is a popular treatment for anxiety and depression that has been used for its medicinal qualities since the Middle Ages. It's the most prescribed anti-depressant in Germany and one of the best-selling herbal remedies in the United States.

Scientifically known as *hypericum perforatum,* the plant is a perennial native to Europe that is now found throughout the U.S. and Canada. Its golden yellow flowers, which bloom in the summer, are said to be at their finest around the June 24th birthday of John the Baptist, for whom it was named.

How it works

St. John's wort is thought to mimic the action of prescription antidepressants, but how it does this is not really known. It is composed of a number of chemicals, and it's not clearly understood which ones are most responsible for its effects. The main herbal components studied have been hypericin and hyperforin.

Research has shown that extracts of some chemicals bind to monoamine oxidase (MAO) types A and B, so it is thought they may act as MAO inhibitors like prescription drugs. However, other research has shown conflicting results.

> When depressive symptoms get in the way of your ability to work, eat, sleep, or enjoy life, it's called major depression. Bipolar disorder — sometimes called manic-depressive — is another serious form of depression. There are also lesser types of depressive disorders.

How effective is it?

During any given year, nearly 10 percent of the population will have some form or intensity of depression. Most research has focused on whether St. John's wort helps reduce the effects of milder forms of this condition.

Reports and studies — mostly from Europe — suggest it works fairly well in these situations. Much of the data, however, has been vague and inconsistent.

Three agencies of the U.S. National Institutes of Health funded a study, using well-defined standards, to see if St. John's wort could help treat moderately severe major depression. The results were that it had no effect on this more serious type of depression.

The study recommended that doctors continue to use proven methods of antidepressant drugs and psychotherapy. But the scientists plan to continue their research to try and establish a level of depression at which St. John's wort can be used effectively.

Problems to watch out for

All St. John's wort products are not the same. Almost all studies use extracts of the hypericum plant rather than the whole herb. Different extracts vary in the amount of hypericin, hyperforin, and other elements they contain.

The U.S. Food and Drug Administration's requirements are less strict for dietary supplements than for regular drugs. The strength and quality of herbal products are unpredictable and can vary from brand to brand and bottle to bottle. It's also possible label information will be misleading or incorrect. You can go online to *www.consumerlab.com* and review their tests to see which supplements have been approved and have the best chance of helping you.

You also need to be concerned about drug interactions. For instance, St. John's wort counteracts certain HIV and anti-cancer drugs. That's one important reason to check with your doctor or pharmacist before taking an herbal remedy. If you already take St. John's wort, be sure and tell your doctor before he treats you for other disorders. The herb can alter the way other medicines work.

MAO inhibitors react with tyramines to produce high blood pressure and stroke. Since it's possible St. John's wort is a MAO inhibitor, stay away from aged cheese, wine, and other foods containing tyramines when taking it.

Quick tips for beating the blahs

Some forms of depression require drug treatment, but often simple changes in behavior or activities are enough to lift that cloud.

- Get regular exercise.
- Listen to music.
- Stop smoking.
- Get enough protein and iron.
- Ask your doctor if a nutritional supplement called SAMe is right for you.
- Eat fish, flaxseed, or walnuts for omega-3 fatty acids.
- Spend time with friends and family.
- Get enough deep, restful sleep.
- Set short-term goals.
- Seek treatment for any health issues.
- Get some sunshine every day.
- Give to others by volunteering.

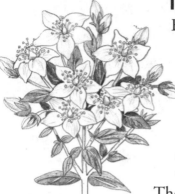

The bottom line

Evidence shows St. John's wort may be useful for treating mild cases of depression, but it's not a proven therapy for more severe depression. If depression is not treated properly, it can get worse and even lead to suicide. It's important to take the right medicines for the proper length of time when dealing with serious depression.

The best course of action is to consult your doctor before taking any drug or herbal remedy. Remember, just because you can buy it over the counter doesn't mean it's safe.

Statins for Alzheimer's

Cholesterol drugs could save your memories

Statins have become the wonder drug of the future, dropping cholesterol like a rock, along with your risk of heart disease — and now possibly Alzheimer's. Scientists are exploring this class of drugs as the next prevention pill for Alzheimer's disease (AD).

If you take them for heart health, you could already be reaping the benefit. But don't break out the champagne yet. There's still work to do.

How it works

Your body can't function without cholesterol, and many cells make it. "It's an important molecule for a lot of things. For instance, cholesterol plays a very important role in how brain cells work and how they respond to injury," explains Dr. Allan

Levey, professor and chairman of the Department of Neurology at Emory University, and director of the Emory Alzheimer's Disease Center. "We know from epidemiologic studies that high cholesterol levels are a risk factor for Alzheimer's disease."

Here's the theory. Amyloid-beta (A-beta) protein builds up in the brains of people with AD. Too much A-beta is believed to be harmful, and scientists believe it contributes to brain damage and eventually death.

This dangerous protein accumulates in a portion of the brain cell called the lipid raft that is important for chemical signaling. Cholesterol seems to play a big role in regulating that compartment, Levey says, so cholesterol helps regulate amyloid-beta levels.

That's where statins join the fight. These drugs lower your cholesterol by limiting how much of it your cells make. "The idea is that by lowering cholesterol levels, we might reduce the amount of beta-amyloid buildup and toxicity that occurs in Alzheimer's disease."

Strong evidence, but more needed

Epidemiological studies have done more than link high cholesterol to AD. They suggest statins could reduce AD risk anywhere from 40 to 70 percent, and that certain ones may help more than others.

Researchers in one such study tracked more than 60,000 seniors. After almost two years, they tallied how many people had developed AD.

- People taking lovastatin, pravastatin, or a combination of these two had the lowest incidence of Alzheimer's disease.

- Suprisingly, simvastatin, another statin drug, did not seem to protect people from AD.

- Non-statin drugs for heart disease also did not help.

A newer epidemiological study suggests statins may offer big rewards in a very short time. After following nearly 3,400 veterans over four years, scientists found:

- those on statins more than a year lowered their AD risk by 29 percent.

- those taking them less than a year dropped it even more, by 44 percent.

- people with high blood pressure, heart disease, or cerebrovascular disease using statins slashed their risk up to 78 percent.

Clinical trials don't paint such a rosy picture. In one placebo-controlled trial of more than 20,000 people, 40 milligrams (mg) of simvastatin a day for five years did not affect people's risk of dementia any more than a placebo.

In a second placebo-controlled trial with 5,800 people, 40 mg of pravastatin each day for three years did not preserve people's mental abilities any better than a placebo.

These differing results do not doom statins for AD. But they don't prove the drugs work, either. "Epidemiologic studies don't show whether something works or not. They show an association," says Levey. "What epidemiologic studies have suggested is very good evidence that people who take statins have a lower risk of Alzheimer's disease.

"Now what these types of studies don't tell you is whether the statin is responsible for reducing that risk," he continues. "For example, the same people who take statins might also be more educated, eat a better diet, exercise more, smoke less, or have lower blood pressure," all factors that lower people's chances of getting Alzheimer's. "You're dealing with a really complicated situation where use of statins may not be the central reason why people have a reduced risk of AD."

Prescription drugs that steal your memory

Even common medications cause side effects, and memory loss could be one of them. Check your medicine cabinet before you blame senility or Alzheimer's, and make sure you're not taking any of these popular drugs. Talk to your doctor about changing your prescription if you suspect it is causing your memory loss.

Disorder	Generic name	Brand name
Anxiety	Alprazolam	Xanax
Depression	Sertraline	Zoloft
High blood pressure	Fosinopril sodium	Monopril
	Lisinopril	Zestril, Prinivil
	Ramipril	Altace
	Amlodipine besylate	Norvasc
	Propranolol hydrochloride	Inderal LA
Sleeping disorders	Zolpidem tartrate	Ambien
Ulcers/GERD	Lansoprazole	Prevacid

Epidemiological studies can point to clues, Levey says, but they can't offer definitive answers. "That's where the clinical trials are important, and those are still ongoing with statins and AD. I don't think we know yet." Experts hope to learn more in the coming years from trials underway now.

Follow this doctor's orders

Levey is hopeful that one day statins could prevent and maybe even treat Alzheimer's — but not yet. If you already take statins for high cholesterol, fine, he says. But don't use them just to protect you from AD. The jury is still out on whether they work, how they work, what dosage you need, and for how long.

"I think there's good reason to be optimistic, but we often get too excited about things," he adds. "We're dealing with a really tough, complicated disease in Alzheimer's, and I'm not sure there will be one wonder drug for it. But statins may be one of many drugs with significant benefits."

If you already use statins, avoid taking them with grapefruit juice, and see your doctor regularly to check for side effects like these:

- nerve damage marked by numbness, pain, or tingling in your hands and feet

- periods of amnesia or extreme memory loss

- liver damage, which your doctor can check with a blood test

You can read more advice on statins and their side effects in the following chapter.

Statins for high cholesterol

★★★

Knock down stubborn LDL

Beating high cholesterol can be tough, but the newest statin drugs lower cholesterol levels better and with fewer side effects than other drugs.

How it works

"Statin drugs will help to lower cholesterol when diet and exercise are not working well enough," explains Mindi Miller, a clinical pharmacist at Emory Healthcare and clinical assistant professor at the University of Georgia College of Pharmacy. You even have six to choose from.

- lovastatin (Mevacor)

- pravastatin (Pravachol)

- fluvastatin (Lescol)

- simvastatin (Zocor)

- atorvastatin (Lipitor)

- rosuvastatin (Crestor)

All the statins block a key substance your liver needs to make cholesterol. "These drugs also help to remove LDL, or bad cholesterol, from the body and can lower triglycerides," Miller says.

Bulldoze more bad cholesterol

According to the National Heart Lung and Blood Institute (NHLBI), studies have reported that people who take statins end up with LDL cholesterol levels that are 20 to 60 percent lower. In addition, a statin might even boost your HDL cholesterol a little. And that's good news because HDL cholesterol helps sweep out LDL.

But two statins may give you more mileage per milligram. Before Crestor came along, research suggested that Lipitor might be the most powerful statin for cutting cholesterol.

But after a six-week study of over 2,000 people with high LDL cholesterol, scientists found that Crestor reduced cholesterol more than three other statins — Lipitor, Zocor, and Pravachol. Crestor lowered LDL by 8 percent more than Lipitor and beat other statins by an even bigger margin.

A new artificial HDL cholesterol may help shave build-up off artery walls. In a small study, those who got weekly intravenous infusions of this HDL had 4 percent less plaque in their arteries after just five weeks. Additional research will determine whether it's safe and effective for everyone. Stay tuned.

Become statin-savvy

Get more out of your statin and help avoid problems with these tips from Miller.

- Avoid grapefruit juice and bypass alcohol.

- Stick with a low-cholesterol, low-fat diet and keep exercising.

- Take the statin with a full glass of water at the same time every day.

- Take your statin two hours before or after antacids, like Mylanta or Maalox.

- Take the statin one hour before or four hours after other cholesterol medicines, like cholestyramine (Questran, Locholest, or Prevalite), colestipol (Colestid), clofibrate (Atromid-S), and fenofibrate (Tricor).

In addition, follow all directions given by your doctor and pharmacist. And talk with your doctor about getting liver function tests periodically while taking statins.

"Statins are well-tolerated by most people," says Miller. But a few of their side effects may be dangerous. Call your doctor right away if you have breathing difficulty, blurred vision, or swelling of the face, tongue, or lips.

Pay less for prescriptions

Get your prescriptions filled without spending a fortune at the pharmacy. Seek discounts online for drugs you use regularly. Shop only at pharmacies that display the VIPPS (Verified Internet Pharmacy Practice Sites) seal. This means a pharmacy is licensed by the states in which it operates and has passed the National Association of Boards of Pharmacy requirements for quality and security. Visit *www.nabp.net* for a list of VIPPS pharmacies.

"Report any muscle pain, tenderness, or weakness, and if you feel different in any way after starting the medication," Miller says, "call your physician immediately." These could be signs of something called statin myopathy — a condition that could lead to kidney damage and other serious problems.

If you're worried that your statin isn't working, remember this. Several studies have shown that statins not only help prevent heart disease they might even reverse some of its progress if you already have it.

"Cardiologists have gone into coronary arteries of patients taking statins and actually documented that fatty buildup has diminished," says Miller. "People will not actually feel different taking statins and may still have chest pain and other symptoms, but rest assured that the medication is working."

Tell your doctor about any other medicines you take. "The statin may cause another medication to work improperly or the other drug may interfere with the statin," says Emory Healthcare clinical pharmacist and University of Georgia professor Mindi Miller. Your doctor can help you avoid dangerous combinations.

Stevia for weight control

FDA nixes natural sweetener

Sugar is the sweetener of choice for many people. Unfortunately, it's full of empty calories. That's why stevia, which is calorie-free and tastes much sweeter than sugar, appeals to folks who want to have their cake — or soft drink — and eat it, too.

How it works

Stevia is an extract that comes from the leaves of a South American shrub. You can use this natural sugar substitute instead of chemical artificial sweeteners, like saccharin and aspartame. Non-nutritive sweeteners make your food and drink taste good, but they don't add the calories found in sugar and high fructose corn syrup.

While it sounds great, stevia has one big drawback. The U.S. Food and Drug Administration (FDA) has not approved it. That means food manufacturers can't put it in drinks, cakes, cookies, candy, or other processed foods.

Although stevia has been widely used in Japan, Korea, and Brazil, the FDA says it doesn't have enough proof to declare it safe. It's also not allowed in Canada and parts of Europe.

Expert says we need to know more

Research on stevia is mixed. Some studies conducted outside the United States say it's OK to use. Other studies suggest there are serious health hazards, like reproductive problems and cancer, especially if it's widely used.

University of Arizona professor emeritus Ryan Huxtable is a toxicologist whose research on stevia is highly regarded by other scientists looking for answers. Huxtable says we don't know enough about it to make a good judgment.

"Its use in other countries is beside the point," he says. "If toxicological associations are not looked for, they will not be found, even if they occur. Consider the use of tobacco for several hundred years by millions of people, without an awareness of associated health problems."

Today, smoking's relationship to cancer and other diseases is obvious, thanks to appropriate research, the professor says.

How big is a serving?		
Item	**Serving size**	**Compare to**
Whole vegetables and fruit	One medium vegetable or piece of fruit	A baseball
Chopped vegetables and fruit	1/2 cup	A rounded handful
Meat	3 ounces	A deck of cards
Rice, mashed potatoes, or pasta	1/2 cup cooked	A tennis ball
Snacks (nuts or pretzels)	1/3 cup	A level handful
Cheese	1 1/2 to 2 ounces	4 dice

Laboratory studies show that stevia could interfere with the way food is converted to energy. That's reason enough to find out what the risk is to humans, Huxtable says. He's also concerned because Americans like sweets a lot more than people in other countries. The amount of stevia used per person in the United States would likely be much more than in Asia or South America.

"Toxicity is a function of dose," he explains. Whether the side effects are worth the benefit from a substance depends on how much of it you use.

Some dangerous reactions might not show up in small-scale studies. A serious public health risk can occur when a product goes on the market and is used by millions of people without careful testing. For example, the arthritis medication Vioxx (rofecoxib) was on the market for five years before a serious association with heart disease was discovered, Huxtable says.

Discover a no-calorie sugar blend

Questions keep popping up about which sugar substitutes are safe to use and which aren't. For example, aspartame may cause headaches, dizziness, and even memory loss. Before you give up on no-calorie sweeteners forever, you might want to consider Sucralose.

Marketed under the name Splenda, it's 600 times sweeter than sugar. Sucralose is made from sugar, so it tastes like sugar. And because it can't be digested, it won't add any calories to your food.

After more than 110 studies performed over 20 years, sucralose was approved for use in 1998.

You'll find it in drinks, snacks, and ice cream. You can also buy it in granular form for use at your table and — since sucralose is heat stable — you can use it in cooking and baking.

Moderation might be the key

Just because something is "natural" doesn't mean it's safe. Until the FDA determines that stevia poses no danger, you won't find it in processed foods as a food additive. However, you can buy it at health food stores and some grocery stores as a dietary supplement. The FDA does not regulate supplements.

Stevia is available as a liquid and a powder. You can buy it in small packets and large cans. Because it's heat resistant, it can be used for baking and cooking, just like regular sugar.

Watchdog groups like the Center for Science in the Public Interest and a United Nations expert panel have concluded that a drop or two in your tea or a little sprinkled on your cereal probably won't be enough to hurt you. But, they don't endorse wide use of this controversial sweetener.

Tea tree oil for insect bites

★ ★ ☆

Soothing relief for skin irritation

Insect bites and other skin irritations can be irritating to say the least. What's more, if you scratch the itching, inflamed, bump they leave behind, you can break your skin and possibly cause yourself more problems. Instead, try using tea tree oil. It can help soothe the itch from the peskiest insects.

How it works

Tea tree oil comes from a native Australian plant. It's a popular herbal remedy for many skin conditions, including insect bites. The swelling that occurs when you get attacked by an insect results from your body's immune system trying to fight off antigens introduced by the bite or sting.

Studies have shown that tea tree oil has antiseptic qualities and may reduce your extra-sensitive response to these allergens and help soothe your inflamed skin. The primary active ingredient in tea tree oil appears to be the water-soluble component terpinen-4-ol.

Reduces inflammation

A recent study involving 27 volunteers tested tea tree oil's anti-inflammatory properties compared to paraffin oil. All volunteers received histamine injections on both forearms, causing inflamed bumps to appear. Tea tree oil was applied to the forearm of 21 volunteers.

The other six volunteers had paraffin oil applied to one of their forearms. Researchers chose liquid paraffin as a control because it's considered the best example of an oil that won't affect your immune system.

As expected, the paraffin oil had no significant effect on the inflamed skin. However, on the 21 volunteers treated with tea tree oil, the inflamed bumps significantly decreased in size by 43 percent an hour after application.

Works on other skin irritations

Tea tree oil works on conditions like scabies as well. In a recent study, tea tree oil was successful at reducing the survival time of the scabies' mites, killing them in just three hours. Researchers believe tea tree oil has the potential to be a new topical treatment against mites.

If you have adult acne, you also may want to try this remedy. A 5-percent tea tree oil gel came out the winner when tested against the popular acne treatment benzoyl peroxide lotion. The tea tree oil reduced breakouts just as effectively as the benzoyl peroxide but with fewer side effects.

Ditch the itch of insect bites

Summer is great, but the insects that come with it are not. Here are some ways to stop the sting and relieve the itch.
- Rub on arnica. It's a natural antibiotic that's safe to use externally.
- Apply half an onion to a bee sting to stop pain and swelling.
- Take the sting out of insect bites with a cold Epsom Salt compress.
- Spread a paste of baking soda and vinegar on bee stings and other insect bites for a soothing sensation.
- Rub some apple cider vinegar on your insect bites.
- Soak mosquito bites in salt water or apply a paste of salt mixed into lard or cold cream.
- Rub jewelweed on mosquito bites.
- Spray insect stings with Fantastik.
- Apply tobacco and snuff juice to wasp stings.

So if you're looking for a treatment without chemicals, look for tea tree oil lotion and soap at your local bath and body shop. You can also find tea tree oil products at your local drug store, herb shop, or health food store.

Don't take internally

Tea tree oil is toxic if swallowed, so be careful. Some products do not have labels warning of their toxicity. One report stated a 4-year-old boy experienced severe muscular and neurological problems within 30 minutes of swallowing a small amount of tea tree oil. Animals, particularly cats, are also susceptible to poisoning.

Tomatoes for heart disease ★★☆

Delicious way to prevent plaque

Whether you like a tangy marinara sauce or a luscious beefsteak tomato fresh off the vine, you may be on the right track to prevent a heart attack.

How it works

The French once called tomatoes love apples. Perhaps that's appropriate because researchers think tomatoes may help prevent heart trouble.

Surprisingly, that trouble may start in your blood vessels. That's where you'll find low density lipoprotein or LDL cholesterol. When unstable molecules — called free radicals — attack LDL particles, the damaged particles become oxidized LDL.

"When LDL is oxidized, it leads to the formation of plaque in the vessel — known as atherosclerosis," explains Dr. Joye

Willcox, a registered dietician and owner of the private weight management practice Healthy Diets, Inc. As more plaques form, the walls of these arteries become thicker, constricting the flow of blood. Eventually, an artery may get clogged enough to cause a heart attack. But that doesn't have to happen.

Willcox and other scientists think something special in tomatoes may help prevent plaque. The most likely candidates may be antioxidants. "Antioxidants provide protection in the inner layer of blood vessels to prevent LDL cholesterol from being oxidized," says Willcox.

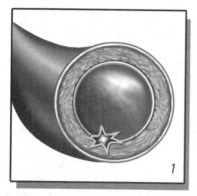

1

Oxidized LDL cholesterol attaches to artery wall. Body recognizes damage and calls for damage control.

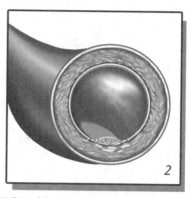

2

White blood cells attach to artery wall. They change into macrophages and eat up all the oxidized LDL nearby, turning them into foam cells.

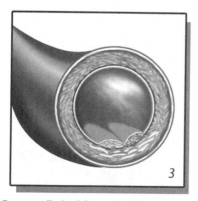

3

Foam cells build up over time, accumulating into fatty streaks.

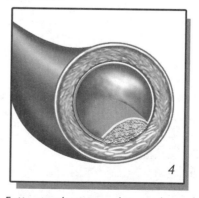

4

Fatty streaks accumulate and plaque forms. As more plaque forms, it begins to clog the artery.

That may mean something as convenient as tomato juice could stop your cholesterol from oxidizing and sticking to your artery walls. You may be able to stop plaque and clogged arteries before they can even get started.

Tomatoes slice risk

Some studies suggest the tomato's most famous antioxidant — lycopene — could be the hero that rescues hearts.

- Dutch researchers examined the blood vessels and blood of 108 elderly people. The higher the amount of lycopene they found in a person's blood, the lower the risk of atherosclerosis seemed to be — especially for smokers or former smokers.

- A study of more than 1,000 men in Finland found those with low levels of lycopene in their blood had thicker artery walls — a sign of atherosclerosis.

- According to American research, older women with more lycopene in their blood may have up to 34 percent less risk of heart disease than those with the lowest lycopene levels.

But Willcox and her colleagues examined the research on what lycopene can do without help from other nutrients. They found some studies where lycopene reduced LDL oxidation and others where it did not. Even studies on other tomato antioxidants had the same mixed results. Yet, research on whole fruits and vegetables consistently showed more promise. Willcox and her colleagues concluded that eating tomatoes and tomato products could be good protection for your heart.

Tomatoes aren't for everyone. If you have heartburn or acid reflux, tomatoes could make your discomfort worse. Some experts also suspect tomatoes may aggravate arthritis.

Cook for a healthier heart

"One cup of tomato sauce or two cups of tomato juice would provide approximately 40 milligrams of lycopene," Willcox says. That amount of daily lycopene from food may be enough to affect the oxidation of LDL cholesterol, according to one study. Another study suggested that drinking 17 ounces of tomato juice every day could do your heart good. But you can also eat your way to lower heart attack risk.

Leading lycopene content in foods

Micrograms of lycopene per 100-gram serving (1/2 cup or 3 1/2 oz. serving)

Food	Lycopene amount
Sun-dried tomatoes	40750
Unsalted tomato paste, canned	28985
Unsalted tomato puree, canned	21754
Ready-to-serve spaghetti sauce	17199
Ketchup	17005
Tomato sauce, canned	15151
Ready-to-serve salsa sauce	10512
Vegetable juice cocktail	9659
Tomato juice with salt added	9037
Tomato soup, canned, prepared with equal volume water	5459
Raw watermelon	4532
Stewed tomatoes, fully ripe and canned	4034
Ripe raw tomato	2572
Raw grapefruit, pink or red	1418

"Cooking appears to increase the absorption of lycopene," says Willcox. That means you may get more lycopene from processed tomato products — especially those with a little oil. For example the oil in tomato paste and tomato sauces helps your body take in more lycopene. For best results, stick with healthy oils like olive oil, and avoid saturated fats and trans fats.

Tums for osteoporosis

Build up your fragile bones

Lack of calcium, the most abundant mineral in your body, is one of the leading nutritional deficiencies in North America today. But there's an easy way to overcome this critical shortfall. Take Tums.

That's right, Tums — the little mint- or fruit-flavored tablet you chew when you have an upset stomach. Tums and many other antacids are made from calcium carbonate because the carbonate neutralizes stomach acid. Carbonate is cheap and easy to find when it's combined with calcium, an important nutrient that can help prevent osteoporosis and a host of other diseases.

In fact, calcium helps your brain and nerve cells work together, and there is even research linking senility and Alzheimer's disease with calcium.

The importance of calcium

"Low calcium intakes have been implicated not just in bone disease, but in obesity, high blood pressure, a variety of cancers — the list is almost so broad it's hard to believe," says Robert P. Heaney, an internationally recognized expert in bone biology and calcium nutrition at Creighton University's Osteoporosis Research Center.

And a brand-new Surgeon General's Report makes a clear statement that there's a huge gap between the amount of calcium Americans take in versus recommended levels.

"Well over half the U.S. public is not getting the calcium intake it ought to have," Heaney, who is both a medical doctor and a professor of medicine, points out. "For certain age ranges, and particularly for women, that could be as much as 85 percent. In a sense, you could just assume you're not getting enough."

There are no outward signs of a simple calcium deficiency. When your body is not taking in enough calcium, it's pulled from your bones to maintain normal nerve and muscle functions. That makes your bones weaker and more likely to break.

The best place to get more calcium is from food, Heaney says. That's because people with low calcium also tend to be low on other nutrients as well. "A low calcium intake is a marker of a poor diet. It's OK to fix that with a calcium supplement, but then you're not fixing the rest of the problem. You need good nutrition on multiple fronts in order to reduce your risk of high blood pressure, obesity, and cancer of the colon and so on," he says.

The primary source of calcium is dairy products. If you aren't drinking at least a couple of glasses of milk a day because you are lactose intolerant, a vegan vegetarian, or some other reason, you might want to take a supplement.

How it works

The calcium carbonate in Tums is the same ingredient used in many tablets sold as calcium supplements. It's effective, cheap, easy to get, and tastes better than other chemical compounds.

You can use other antacids, but be sure and check the ingredients. Other substances, like magnesium carbonate and aluminum hydroxide gel, might actually be better antacids, but unless the antacid contains calcium, it won't help your bones.

Delicious ways to get more calcium		
Food	Serving size	Milligrams of calcium
Yogurt, plain, low-fat	8 oz.	415
Sardines, canned in oil, with bones	3 oz.	324
Milk, non-fat	1 cup	302
Milk, whole	1 cup	291
Mozzarella, part-skim	1 1/2 oz.	275
Spinach, cooked	1/2 cup	120
Ice cream, vanilla	1/2 cup	85
Broccoli, raw	1/2 cup	21
Bread, whole wheat	1 slice	20

You get the best results when you chew a single 400 or 500 milligram (mg) tablet two or three times a day. That's because calcium isn't easily absorbed, and absorption goes down when you take larger doses.

However, Heaney says it doesn't hurt to take a large dose, like 1,000 mg, because the more you take in, the more you absorb. For instance, you may absorb 30 percent of a 100 mg dose, but only 15 percent of 1,000 mg. That's still 150 mg against only 30 mg from the more efficient dose.

How much do you need?

"You probably need to absorb a couple hundred milligrams of calcium a day," advises Heaney. That means taking in 1,000 to 1,500 mg.

This is particularly important with older people because calcium absorption drops off as you age. Calcium absorption can be as high as 60 percent in babies and young children, but it slowly drops to 15 to 20 percent in adulthood. After age 50, it's even lower.

Other factors that increase risk for osteoporosis and the need for calcium include being female, thin, or inactive, smoking, and excessive use of alcohol. It's also more important for postmenopausal women to get enough calcium because the lack of estrogen increases bone loss.

Just don't overdo it. The Tolerable Upper Intake Level for calcium is 2,500 mg a day, so consider your entire dietary

Dynamic duo — vitamin D and calcium

Chances are you're not getting enough vitamin D, the nutrient that helps your body absorb calcium and keeps your bones strong. Here's how you can get more:

- Eat cold-water fish, like salmon, sardines, and herring.
- Eat vitamin D-fortified foods, such as ready-to-eat cereals, milk, and other dairy products.
- Eat an egg occasionally. There's vitamin D in the yolk.
- Get a little sun. Your body can easily make vitamin D from the sun's ultraviolet rays. Experts recommend 10 to 15 minutes of sunlight — without wearing sunscreen — twice a week on your face, hands, and legs. If you stay out in the sun longer, apply a sunscreen with an SPF of at least 15.

Unfortunately, as you age, your digestive system's ability to absorb vitamin D from food and your skin's ability to convert sunlight to vitamin D decline.

If you think you are at risk for a deficiency, check with your doctor about taking supplements. Just remember — too much vitamin D from supplements can be toxic.

intake — including fortified foods — before adding supplements. Check with your doctor or a registered dietician for help in figuring out your exact needs. The Recommended Adequate Intake for adults 51 years or older is 1,200 mg.

Too much calcium can cause kidney problems and interfere with the absorption of other minerals in your body. Other side effects include gas, bloating, and constipation. If side effects are a problem for you, take your supplement with meals.

There are many types and brands of calcium supplements and Heaney's research has shown that not all are manufactured as well as others. If you're not happy with the one you are taking, try a different one.

Vegetarian diet for colon cancer

★★★

Cut cancer risk with plant-based foods

A vegetarian diet is a good way to protect yourself from colorectal cancer, the third-most common cancer for both men and women.

When you eat a lot of fat and red meat and not very many fruits, vegetables, and whole grains, your risk of colon cancer increases. Of course, a vegetarian diet won't guarantee you'll never get cancer, but it's like not smoking — a healthy choice.

Vegetarianism isn't complicated. It's simply the practice of eating foods that come from plants. You don't even have to swear off meat completely, although many people do.

How it works

Colorectal cancer starts from tiny stemlike growths inside your colon called polyps. These polyps usually start out as non-cancerous and show up more often in people who eat a lot of meat and not many plant-based foods.

Scientists talk a lot about whether eating meat causes colon cancer or if eating fruit, vegetables, and whole grains stops it. The only clear answer is you need to both lower your meat and fat intake and increase the amount of plant-based foods in your diet. Here's why.

Colon polyps seem to grow more profusely when there are fecal bile acids around. These are acids secreted by your liver to help digest fats in your intestines. A high meat diet, full of saturated fat, naturally produces more fecal bile acids. And so, you increase your risk of polyps the more red meat you eat.

- One recent study, done in Singapore, found Chinese women eating the most meat and least vegetables were more than twice as likely to develop colorectal cancer.

Cabbage crushes cancer

The next time you're cruising the produce aisles, stock up on this cheap, low-calorie, proven cancer-crusher. Studies from around the world show cabbage guards you not only from colon cancer, but breast, brain, bladder, stomach, and lung cancers as well.

Cabbage belongs to the cruciferous family of vegetables, which includes broccoli, cauliflower, turnips, and brussels sprouts. They all have high cancer-fighting nutrients.

Eat cabbage raw or only lightly cooked for the most cancer protection. Slaw can be a welcome alternative to the traditional dinner salad, or for an ethnic treat, try corned beef and cabbage (Irish), sauerkraut (German), or kimchi (Korean).

Top sources of fiber	
Food	**Grams of fiber per cup**
Barley, pearled, raw	31.2
Bulgur, dry	25.6
Navy beans, boiled	19.1
Red kidney beans, canned	16.4
Split peas, boiled	16.3
Lentils, boiled	15.6
Pinto beans, boiled	15.4
Black beans, boiled	15.0
Wheat flour, whole-grain	14.6
Oat bran, raw	14.5
Dates, deglet noor	14.2
Refried beans, canned	13.4
Lima beans, large, boiled	13.2

The nutrients and phytochemicals in fruits and vegetables play an important role — vitamin D, folate, and antioxidants are all proven cancer fighters — but dietary fiber may be the biggest reason a vegetarian diet foils colon cancer.

Experts believe fiber grabs on to potential cancers in your digestive system and carries them out of your body with waste material. Fiber also encourages a process in your lower intestine that gets rid of those dangerous fecal bile acids that promote polyps.

- One important study that focused on dietary fiber, researched almost 520,000 people from 10 different countries in Europe. They found when people increased their daily intake of fiber from approximately 15 to 35 grams, they lowered their colon cancer risk by 40 percent.

Some starches are indigestible and act like fiber against bile acids and carcinogens in the large intestine. Called resistant starches, these are found in unprocessed legumes like black beans, kidney beans, lentils, and peas; and unprocessed cereal grains such as corn, sorghum, and barley.

"5-a-day" now minimum for benefit

Five servings per day used to be the accepted standard for fruits and vegetables. But now a group that includes the National Cancer Institute and the American Cancer Society says that

---

Virtual colonoscopy gets lukewarm reviews

A colonoscopy without that uncomfortable viewing tube inserted in your rectum — sounds great, right? Not necessarily, says a Johns Hopkins educational report.

Called a virtual colonoscopy, this procedure uses a computed tomography (CT) scan or magnetic resonance imaging (MRI) to check your colon for cancer-causing polyps. Not a tube in sight.

There are, however, some drawbacks.

- You still have to undergo the same bowel-cleansing routine before the procedure.
- Air is pumped into your colon to distend it, which can cause painful cramping.
- You won't receive any sedatives.
- You'll still need a traditional colonoscopy to remove any polyps they find.
- Virtual colonoscopies often miss or misdiagnose polyps.
- Most insurance plans won't pay for the procedure.

should only be a minimum. Active women need seven servings a day; active men need nine.

Add some whole grains to that and you'll probably eat less meat without even trying — there won't be room on your plate or in your stomach.

You may be closer to these recommendations than you think. A serving is only about as much as will fit in the palm of your hand. That's a medium stalk of broccoli, a half-dozen baby carrots, or a small banana. Other single servings are:

- one-half cup of cooked vegetables, diced fruit or vegetables, or cooked beans
- one-fourth cup of dried fruit
- a full cup of raw salad greens
- 6 ounces of 100 percent fruit or vegetable juice

Vitamin C for atherosclerosis

★★☆

Eat your way to healthy arteries

Frankie Ford scored a top-20 hit in 1959 with the song "Sea Cruise." Follow his advice, and you'll have smooth sailing when it comes to your arteries. Just take yourself on a "C" cruise. Vitamin C could be a smash hit in the battle against atherosclerosis.

How it works

Experts who say vitamin C can help clean your arteries have based their theories in part on vitamin C's valuable role as an antioxidant. Researchers theorize that vitamin C helps keep low-density lipoproteins (LDL, the "bad" cholesterol) from oxidizing, which helps protect the arteries in your heart and brain from getting clogged.

This vitamin also strengthens your blood vessel walls, which promotes good circulation. Some studies also show vitamin C can prevent blood vessels from constricting and cutting off blood flow to your heart and brain.

Stick with fresh fruits and vegetables, though. Recent research has shown that antioxidant supplements have little or no proven value in heading off heart disease.

Boost vitamin C to lower risk

While the evidence is not rock-solid, vitamin C seems to help your heart and arteries in a number of ways.

Nutritional powerhouses attack atherosclerosis

You can help prevent the clogged arteries and poor circulation of atherosclerosis with a simple combination of vitamins and minerals. These vitamins even help stop cataracts.

- Vitamin E guards your arteries from plaque build-up. Eat wheat germ, vegetable oils, nuts, seeds, and leafy green vegetables.
- Use vitamin C to neutralize toxic chemicals, called free radicals, that cause your arteries to harden. Good sources include citrus fruits, broccoli, red and green peppers, and strawberries. An added bonus — vitamin C protects your eyes against damaging free radicals that can cause cataracts.
- Folate, a B vitamin, helps your blood vessels dilate, or widen, so more blood and oxygen can get through. So pile on the dark leafy greens, legumes, and enriched breads and cereals.
- Potassium, magnesium, and calcium all work to lower your blood pressure, a major factor in developing atherosclerosis. Eat a variety of fruits, vegetables, and dairy foods for these important minerals.

- A Korean study found people who had the highest intake of vitamin C slashed their risk of heart disease by two-thirds compared to those who got the least.

- Researchers in Scotland reported vitamin C reduced arterial stiffness in healthy people, while a Finnish study showed vitamin C, along with vitamin E, helped slow the progression of atherosclerosis.

- Japanese scientists determined that high concentrations of vitamin C in your blood may significantly reduce your risk for stroke. A Dutch study also found high vitamin C intake may lower your stroke risk.

- Vitamin C helps lower blood pressure in older people, according to a study in the UK.

- Arizona State University researchers showed that orange juice helps thwart lipids, or fats, in your blood. A glassful of this with your meals can fight heart-damaging free radicals. You can also find low-calorie orange juice or orange juice fortified with plant sterols to help lower cholesterol.

Not all results are positive. Several studies showed vitamin C offered neither harm nor help.

Focus on foods

The Recommended Dietary Allowance (RDA) of vitamin C is 90 mg for men and 75 mg for women, but you can safely get up to 2,000 mg per day.

It's easy to get enough vitamin C through your diet. It's also better for you. With vitamin C supplements, you can get too much of a good thing. Too much vitamin C can lead to bloating and diarrhea. It may also cause you to absorb too much iron, lead to kidney stones, or erode the enamel on your teeth.

10 super sources of 'C'

Wondering where to find the most vitamin C? Look no further than these 10 foods that clean and flush out your arteries.

Sweet red pepper	226 mg
Papaya	188 mg
Broccoli, 1 cup cooked	101 mg
Strawberries, 1 cup	98 mg
Brussels sprouts, 1 cup cooked	97 mg
Green pepper	96 mg
Cranberry juice cocktail	90 mg
Orange juice, 1 cup chilled	82 mg
Kiwi fruit	71 mg
Orange	70 mg

Instead of supplementing, stick to vitamin C-rich foods. Besides vitamin C, whole foods also give you fiber and other nutrients that help fight atherosclerosis.

You don't have to stick to tried and true sources of vitamin C, either. Have fun finding unusual — and tasty — ways to get more of this important vitamin. For example, try a delicious fruit that keeps your arteries open for business. Who says you have to rely only on blood thinning drugs? Consider eating a persimmon instead, a reddish-orange fruit packed with fiber, potassium, magnesium, calcium and antioxidants, all super weapons for fighting atherosclerosis.

Or eat a papaya, a tropical fruit with more than twice the vitamin C of an orange. It also gives you plenty of potassium, folate, and fiber to protect you from heart attack and stroke.

Just be careful if you take the blood-thinning medication warfarin. A compound in papayas called papain may make its effects stronger.

Enjoy your "C" cruise — it just might be a permanent vacation from atherosclerosis. Bon voyage!

Walking for high blood pressure

Simple steps to healthy arteries

Spring is here. Time to start watering the lawn again. Fred screws the hose to the spigot and turns on the H_2O. To his amazement, water starts squirting from leaks along the whole length of the hose. Months of neglect have taken their toll. The old hose can't take the pressure any more.

So it is with untreated high blood pressure. The fix may not be as simple as running to the garden shop for a new hose, but walking there, instead of driving, is a good way to start.

How it works

The garden hose helps explain how blood pressure works. Pressure in the hose increases as the faucet opens or as the nozzle is twisted to reduce flow.

In the same way, blood pressure depends on the volume of blood being pumped by your heart and the resistance to the flow in the small arteries.

High blood pressure is a sign that your heart is working too hard — usually because of a blockage or inflexibility in the "hoses." Those small arteries have muscle fibers in their walls that are supposed to constrict and dilate, giving vessels some healthy flexibility. High blood pressure lets you know the flex is gone. If not controlled, heart disease and other serious health problems aren't far off.

Walking reconditions your arteries. And there's a bonus. It reduces your risk of heart attack and stroke and improves the quality of your life while adding extra active years.

When you walk, your heart beats harder and your blood pressure temporarily rises because your muscles need more blood. But once your heart and blood vessels get in shape, they won't need to work so hard to do their job, and your blood pressure will drop.

By walking, you'll get your blood pressure in the healthy range and keep it there without dangerous drugs or overly strenuous exercise.

Warning signs of a heart attack

Do you know the nine signs that a heart attack is in progress or about to begin? If you have high blood pressure, this wisdom is essential for every member of your family. Knowing these signs can mean the difference between life and death. When in doubt, call 911.

- Chest pain or discomfort, like uncomfortable pressure, squeezing, tightness, or fullness, that lasts more than a few minutes — or it may go away and return.
- Pain or discomfort spreading to shoulders, arms, or other parts of your upper body, like jaw, neck, stomach, or back.
- Shortness of breath, with or without chest discomfort.
- A cold sweat, even in cool weather.
- Unexplainable weakness, lightheadedness, dizziness, or fatigue.
- Nausea, indigestion, or gas-like pain.

Research proves benefits of walking

Recent studies show that a 30-minute brisk walk each day can dramatically lower your blood pressure, as well as help you lose weight, reduce stress, and treat diabetes by reducing your need for insulin or drugs.

Researchers, reviewing the results of more than 50 studies, kept track of the blood pressure of nearly 2,500 previously sedentary adults. Walking briskly for 30 minutes every day led to an average drop of 3.8 in systolic blood pressure, the top number, and 2.6 in the diastolic, the number on the bottom.

These decreases translate into a huge drop in heart disease and heart attacks. What's more, walking itself is safer than more rigorous exercise for those with high blood pressure and heart disease — and more effective than relying solely on medication or diet.

What's more, if 30 minutes seems too much, this research shows you'll get positive results even if you walk in 10-minute increments throughout the day.

> People with high blood pressure are in greater jeopardy for suffering heart attacks when winter arrives. Cold weather causes blood vessels to narrow, restricting blood flow, which increases blood pressure. What's more, the risk soars when temperatures drop by as little as nine degrees in a day — even if it's not chilly. The best defense? Dress warmly when going out in the cold.

Another study found that gravity affects your blood pressure. Russian researchers examining the effects of spaceflight found that the gravitational stress of prolonged sitting results in high blood pressure. Who's most likely to suffer this downside of gravity? Not astronauts, but couch potatoes.

So if couch potato describes you, get up and take a walk before your blood pressure goes into orbit. Just think. You can

Walking plan: 45 minutes in 12 weeks				
	Warm Up	**Brisk Walk**	**Cool Down**	**Total Time**
Week 1	5 min	5 min	5 min	15 min
Week 2	5 min	7 min	5 min	17 min
Week 3	5 min	9 min	5 min	19 min
Week 4	5 min	11 min	5 min	21 min
Week 5	5 min	13 min	5 min	23 min
Week 6	5 min	15 min	5 min	25 min
Week 7	5 min	18 min	5 min	28 min
Week 8	5 min	21 min	5 min	31 min
Week 9	5 min	24 min	5 min	34 min
Week 10	5 min	27 min	5 min	37 min
Week 11	5 min	31 min	5 min	41 min
Week 12	5 min	35 min	5 min	45 min

talk, laugh, and sing whether you're sitting or walking. The difference is, sitting raises blood pressure, walking lowers it.

Tell high blood pressure to take a hike

The path to lower blood pressure begins with steps as simple as using stairs instead of elevators, parking at the far end of the lot, or getting off the bus a block early.

If unassisted walking is tough for you, the National Heart, Lung, and Blood Institute offers some options.

- wheel yourself in a wheelchair 30 to 40 minutes
- push a stroller a mile and a half in 30 minutes

- swim laps 20 minutes or do water aerobics for 30

Check with your doctor first if you already have heart disease, are over 50 and not used to physical activity, have a family history of heart disease at an early age, or have other health problems.

Water for weight loss

Burn calories the easy way

What a splash it would make if you could effectively lose weight by drinking lots of water. Some people are giving it a try and swearing by it. But until further research comes in, swimming is still the best water-based weight-loss regimen around.

How it works

Health and nutrition textbooks are a wellspring of information on the importance of water to your body. It transports nutrients, cleanses cells, carries away waste, lubricates joints, cushions organs, and regulates body temperature. Drinking eight to 10 glasses a day is a healthy habit, but will it also help you lose weight?

Some experts say drinking lots of water will make you feel full, so you'll be less likely to overeat. Others say water may help clear wastes from your body more efficiently.

But research points to a possible effect on metabolism as the key to water's value in weight loss. Drinking a lot of water may actually

> Unlike what you may have heard, soda, coffee, tea, and other caffeinated beverages count toward your daily water total, according to Dr. Heinz Valtin, researcher and professor emeritus at Dartmouth Medical School.

raise your metabolic rate, which is the rate at which you burn calories. In one study, drinking cold water after a meal led to an increase in fat burning in men, while in women, drinking water increased carbohydrate burning.

The jury is still out on whether water truly has an impact on weight loss, but scientists do agree it provides great benefits to your body, so it can't hurt to try. When it comes to managing your weight, every little health improvement can be significant.

Water's benefits weigh in

One study by scientists in Germany and Canada looked at the influence of drinking water on metabolism. Their findings suggest water increases your metabolic rate within 10 minutes of drinking it and lasts for an hour or more.

They found that drinking 1.5 liters (6 cups) of water each day could help you burn 48 more calories. That adds up to 17,400 calories per year or about 5 pounds!

Nevertheless, reviews of this research are mixed. Some suggest the study was too small — only 14 subjects. Other critics claim the additional calories burned by drinking extra water won't necessarily translate into noticeable weight loss. Of course, if your daily water replaces high-calorie sodas and other beverages, that could be a different story.

Delicious sources of water	
Food	**Water content by weight**
1 head of iceberg lettuce	95 percent
1 large cucumber unpeeled	95 percent
1 wedge of watermelon	91 percent
1 raw papaya	88 percent

Don't overlook water "supplements" in your weight-loss program, either. Many fresh fruits and vegetables are 80 to 99 percent water as well as natural great-tasting sources of this healthful liquid. Try cucumbers, lettuce, summer squash, watermelon, grapefruit, strawberries, apples, and tomatoes for the most water-dense additions to your diet.

Wristband for motion sickness

★★☆

Steady pressure calms nausea

A simple, inexpensive solution to motion sickness is at hand — literally. A special band you wear around your wrist could quell those uncomfortable symptoms that ruin your car, boat, and plane trips.

Experts claim acupressure wristbands not only relieve motion sickness but other sick-to-your-stomach feelings as well. They've been used to prevent nausea and vomiting from surgical anesthesia, pregnancy, and chemotherapy.

How it works

Motion sickness happens when your ears sense your body is moving, but your eyes don't think it is. Reading in the car is a good example. You can also get sick from the opposite effect — when your body is stationary, but your eyes are picking up movement. Symptoms may include headache, nausea, and vomiting.

Using a wristband to control nausea may sound strange, but it's based on the ancient Chinese principle of acupressure, a needleless form of acupuncture. In traditional Chinese medicine, the area about 2 inches above the inner wrist, known as the Neiguan or Pericardium 6 (P6) point, is associated with nausea and vomiting.

Applying pressure to a meridian point associated with a certain area of the body is thought to relieve the pain or discomfort occurring there. By using a wristband to apply continuous pressure to the P6 point, you may find relief from the uncomfortable symptoms of motion sickness.

Positive results

A study at Pennsylvania State University had 25 people look at moving black and white stripes to bring about motion sickness. Each subject went through three sessions — one with a wristband on the P6 location, one with it further up their arm, and one with no wristband at all.

Seventy-two percent of the subjects reported less motion sickness when they wore the wristbands in the proper position. However, 64 percent were better by just having the band on their forearm. The researchers noted that the secondary location might have stimulated nerves that connected to the same network as the P6 location did.

It's also possible that a placebo effect causes people to feel better just because they think they are going to. Doctors at the University of Rochester in New York did a random wristband test on 739 chemotherapy patients. They found that people who expected the wristbands to work got more relief than those who didn't.

The Rochester study also showed patients using acupressure bands had less nausea and vomiting on the day of the treatment than those who didn't. During the five days following treatment, the wristbands didn't seem to make any difference.

A study at a Brooklyn hospital found wristbands reduced post-operative sickness significantly. It noted that the bands were much cheaper than drugs, had virtually no side effects, and that patients liked them better than drugs.

Find the right kind

You can buy wristbands at drug stores and through the Internet for about $10 a pair. Some brands are made of Velcro so they can be adjusted to the exact size of your wrist. Others depend on elastic to provide the pressure.

But they all use a round plastic bead to stimulate the pressure point on your wrist. After attaching the band, rub or push on the bead for several moments to help start the therapeutic effect.

Fancier wristbands deliver a battery-powered electrical stimulus instead of using pressure. But it's best to start off with the less-expensive bands to see whether they work for you first.

Ginger soothes the savage beast

This ancient natural cure tops the list of stomach soothers. Try it — or these other remedies — to ward off motion sickness.

Ginger, half an hour before traveling, should prevent the symptoms of motion sickness. You'll find it at any supermarket or health food store. A typical capsule, containing 500 milligrams (mg) of ginger, is usually enough to quiet your gastrointestinal tract. But some herbal experts recommend taking two. Repeat as symptoms develop.

Candied ginger is another way to enjoy ginger's benefits. See if your grocery store carries this sweet treat, or check an Oriental market. A 1-inch square equals the amount of ginger in one 500-mg capsule.

And if you can find it, naturally flavored ginger ale — not the artificial kind — has been used for years to calm nausea.

Otherwise, suck on a lemon, nibble soda crackers, relax, avoid overeating, breathe fresh air, don't smoke, and don't drink alcohol.

Yoga for asthma

Avoid attacks with exercise

You can take the fright out of an asthma attack with a remedy that's as old as the hills. Yoga, which means "united" or "joined together," is actually several disciplines united to make body and mind work in harmony.

Since its introduction to the Western world, yoga has become more user-friendly to Americans and Europeans. It's even being touted to relieve symptoms of chronic health problems, like asthma. This is great news since the World Health Organization estimates asthma afflicts more than 100 million people worldwide.

How it works

Yoga may be the ideal workout for people with asthma. Many asthmatics avoid exercise because of the fear of suffering an attack. But the slow, controlled movements and deep breathing of yoga promotes relaxation while relieving stiffness and limbering up the body.

The breathing exercises that are essential to this exercise program not only open up the lungs but may possibly reduce the inflammation that occurs with asthma.

Some researchers also think the relaxation/meditation aspect of yoga could help asthmatics by regulating breathing patterns and improving lung function. Easing your symptoms through yoga is one positive way to help manage your condition.

Science meets yoga

Researchers are still looking for answers. In one long-term study, 106 people with asthma were divided into two groups.

One group practiced yoga breathing techniques, while the other group served as the control. Researchers discovered that the people practicing yoga required less asthma medication and suffered fewer asthma attacks during the study.

Another trial tested a yoga meditation technique called Sahaja. Participants sought to reach a state of "mental silence." They were alert and aware but free of any unnecessary mental activity.

Researchers found that the people using Sahaja also succeeded in reducing their asthma medication. During the four-month test period, the average number of acute attacks for meditators was 5.8, compared to 12.9 for the control group.

Get out of your rut

People with asthma who hesitate to exercise, whose shoulders are stooped from shallow breathing, and whose general health and outlook on life have been suffocated by asthma could benefit from yoga.

It typically involves three aspects. They often overlap and complement one another.

- Hatha yoga — gradual, gentle movements and poses called asanas. Hatha yoga strengthens and invigorates your body and lungs.

- Pranayama — the exercise of controlled breathing. Prana means "breath of life."

- Meditation — exercise for the will. Meditation helps you get a handle on stress and worry and regain a hopeful outlook about your health.

If you decide to practice yoga, find a reputable instructor because doing the techniques improperly may result in injury.

To find a yoga instructor in your area, contact your local recreation department, YMCA, or fitness center.

While yoga won't eliminate your asthma, it might help you control your symptoms. Talk with your doctor about using it as a complement to traditional treatments.

---

8 tricks for better breathing

- Drink lots of water to keep your airways moist.
- Take ginkgo biloba, an herbal supplement that can prevent bronchospasms — a sudden narrowing in your air passages. Experts recommend 40 milligrams of ginkgo three times a day.
- Get some omega-3 fatty acids every week from foods like salmon, herring, halibut, wheat germ, and walnuts.
- Find out if you suffer from GERD (gastroesophageal reflux disease) and treat it. There is a link between this condition and asthma.
- Learn to breathe better. That means taking slow, deep, full breaths in through your nose and expelling all the air when you breathe out.
- Maintain a healthy weight through good diet and exercise.
- Take a 30-second cold shower every day to improve breathing.
- If your asthma is based on an allergy — to mold, dust, animals, etc. — control your condition by removing these triggers from your environment.

Yoga for weight loss

★★☆

Speed up your metabolism

Yoga is an easy way to lose weight and rejuvenate your metabolism. When your metabolism is revved up, you automatically burn more fat.

The yoga approach to weight loss involves both physical and mental exercises — boosting your self-confidence and strengthening your self-control.

How it works

You may not think yoga is strenuous enough to help you lose weight, but it's a lot more challenging than it looks. This ancient art helps you build strength and flexibility and works on your aerobic conditioning, breathing, and relaxation.

In fact, this total body-mind focus is the key to its success in weight management. By embracing the "holistic" mindset of all-around good health, which includes reaching and maintaining a healthy weight, you incorporate a positive image into all aspects of your life.

Yoga is a program that helps you cultivate realistic goals and expectations, rather than a get-thin-quick mindset that focuses on killer exercises and fad dieting. It helps you understand why you're overweight and provides a means of addressing those issues through exercise and relaxation.

The traditional poses can be done at your own pace, either alone or with a group, and this flexibility is an incentive to stick with the program. The deep breathing and slow movements help relieve stress and provide you with renewed energy. Once you incorporate yoga into your life, you'll wonder how you ever managed without it.

Study shows more pounds lost

A study conducted by the University of Pittsburgh shows that yoga can help you lose weight. A group of 59 obese, inactive women were placed on a low-fat diet and assigned to either walk, walk and do strength-training exercises, or walk and do yoga.

After four months, those who only walked had lost an average of 20 pounds. Those who walked and did strength-training exercises had lost an average of 23 pounds. And those who walked and did yoga had lost an average of 27 pounds.

Take a class to do it right

Since yoga is a precise discipline, its postures and breathing techniques must be done correctly to prevent injury or hyperventilation. Contact your community recreation center or a nearby hospital for information about yoga classes in your area.

Learning this ancient art might help you rediscover the healthy pleasure of being in control of your body, your diet, your exercise habits, and your ability to relax and enjoy life.

Zinc for colds

Relief from annoying symptoms

Colds are responsible for at least 62 million doctors' visits every year. That's why scientists have been searching for centuries to find a cure.

While zinc may not be a miracle cure, it might provide quicker relief from symptoms or help keep you from getting a cold in the first place.

How it works

Your body contains a small amount of zinc. This trace mineral works with proteins in every organ and helps enzymes do their jobs.

And that's not all — getting enough of this vital nutrient keeps your immune system healthy. A strong immune system protects you from infections and viruses — like colds and flu.

People with low zinc levels have fewer T-cells, which identify and destroy harmful substances in your body, like bacteria and viruses. Not having enough T-cells increases your susceptibility to infections. When people with a zinc deficiency raise their zinc levels, T-cell levels increase as well.

Foils viruses two ways

Research on the effectiveness of zinc for colds falls into two categories — the study of topical treatments, like lozenges and nasal sprays and gels, for those who already have a cold, and the study of how getting enough in your diet influences your health.

Some studies show that zinc whips colds, but others aren't so favorable. Several factors seem to influence the results, like the form of zinc you take (zinc gluconate, zinc acetate, zinc sulfate, zinc citrate, or zinc picolinate), how much you take, how you take it (topically or as a supplement), and whether or not those who were studied had a zinc deficiency to begin with.

You don't take topical treatments to increase your body's zinc level. You use them to interfere with viruses in your nose and throat where colds begin. Numerous studies on the effectiveness of topical zinc have shown positive results, as long as zinc gluconate or acetate is used — the best results coming from zinc gluconate. Zinc sulfate hasn't done so well in those tests.

In one study, 213 people just coming down with a cold used one squirt of a zinc gluconate nasal gel or placebo in each nostril every four hours during the day. The people who used the zinc nasal gel recovered in about two days, compared to nine days for those using the placebo.

According to another study, if you take zinc at the first sign of colds or flu, your symptoms may be gone within 24 hours.

Other studies involved zinc's influence on the immune system. Researchers discovered that consuming extra zinc during the cold and flu season actually helps prevent illness. People who took zinc supplements during the cold and flu season came down with fewer colds than those who didn't.

Zinc cautions

It's not difficult to get enough zinc from the food you eat. If you like to eat oysters, you should be getting plenty of zinc. Not an oyster lover? Zinc is also found in other seafood, as well as red meat, poultry, legumes, and whole grains.

However, if you're one of the estimated 90 percent of healthy elderly people who don't get enough zinc, supplements may be the answer.

Before deciding to supplement with zinc, consider how much you are getting in your diet. You can get too much zinc. In

---

Extraordinary tea soothes sore throat

Few things hurt as much as a sore throat. And few remedies do much to help — except Throat Coat.

Throat Coat is an herbal tea made of ingredients traditionally used for throat health. It aids vocal cords so you can speak, esophagus so you can swallow, and trachea so you can breathe easier.

Throat Coat's ingredients include:

- althea root and slippery elm bark, which create a protective coating for your throat
- licorice root, known for quieting coughs and soothing inflamed tissue
- marshmallow root, which relieves dry cough irritation

The tea's naturally sweet taste makes it enjoyable for everyone from children to singers or anyone else seeking relief.

For doubters, Throat Coat endured the scrutiny of a double-blind, placebo-controlled trial and came through with flying colors. It really works!

fact, consuming more than you need can impair your immunity, irritate your stomach, and cause vomiting and other serious side effects. The Recommended Dietary Allowance for men age 51 or older is 11 milligrams a day. For women age 51 or older, it's 8 mg.

Zinc supplements combine elemental zinc with other substances. When choosing a supplement, check the amount of elemental zinc listed on the label, since that's what your body uses. An 80-mg supplement of zinc gluconate might contain only 10 mg of elemental zinc.

To relieve sore throats and other cold symptoms, many experts say it's safe to use zinc lozenges — sparingly. Don't overdo it. Some people take higher and higher doses to achieve relief, which could cause a zinc overdose.

When buying lozenges, look for a form of zinc called zinc gluconate glycine, which is easily released when you suck on the lozenge.

Sources

8 Steps to a Healthy Heart, Warner Books, New York, 1994

A

About air cleaners, Clean Air Delivery Rate, American Home Appliance Manufacturers <http://cadr.org/consumer/index.html> retrieved Jan. 12, 2005

Acupuncture, Arthritis Today Online, The Arthritis Foundation <www.arthritis.org> retrieved September 8, 2004

Advances in Therapy (18,4:189; 20,4:220; and 21,2:61)

Ageing Research Reviews (2,1:1)

Alcohol Alert, National Institute on Alcohol Abuse and Alcoholism <www.niaaa.nih.gov> retrieved Oct. 24, 2004

Alcohol Research and Health (25,2:101)

Alimentary Pharmacology & Therapeutics (13,8:1103; 16,12:2029; and 18,11:1113)

Alive: Canadian Journal of Health and Nutrition, May 2004

Allan Levey, M.D., professor and chairman of the Department of Neurology at Emory University and director of the Emory Alzheimer's Disease Center, Atlanta

Alternative & Complementary Therapies (5,4:199 and 5,5:266)

Alternative and Complementary Medicine (9,2:285)

Alternative Medical Review (3,4:308; 4,6:392; and 6,4:383)

Alternative Therapies – Glucosamine and Chrondroitin Sulfate, The Arthritis Foundation <www.arthritis.org> retrieved Oct. 29, 2004

Alternative Therapies (6,3:61,62)

Alternative Therapies in Health and Medicine (7,4:91 and 10,2:36)

American Chemical Society news release (Sept. 18, 2002)

American Family Physician (58,8:1795; 68,5:923; 68,8:1539; 70,1:133; and 70,11:2175)

American Heart Association. Heart Disease and Stroke Statistics — 2004 Update, American Heart Association, Dallas, Texas, 2003

American Heart Journal (147,3:401)

American Journal of Cardiology (90,10:1150; 91,11:1316; and 92,2:152)

American Journal of Clinical Dermatology (1,6:369)

American Journal of Clinical Nutrition (51,6:1013; 67,1:136; 70,3:504S; 70,4:466; 71,2:472; 73,6:1010; 76,1:148; 77,1:133; 77,2:281; 77,3:532; 78,3:544S; 78,3:647S; 78,5:920; 79,6:1020; 80,1:123; 80,2:245; 80,2:396; and 80,5:1358)

American Journal of Gastroenterology (98,2:348)

American Journal of Health-System Pharmacies (60,13:1310)

American Journal of Medicine (116,2:91)

American Journal of Therapeutics (10,5:324)

American Tinnitus Association <www.ata.org> retrieved Dec. 7, 2004

Anesthesia and Analgesia (84,4:821 and 94,6:1639)

Angiotensin-converting Enzyme (ACE) Inhibitors (Systemic), MedlinePlus <www.nlm.nih.gov> retrieved Nov. 1, 2004

Annals of Internal Medicine (136,1:42; 136,7:493; 137,12:939; 139,9:724; 140,1:1; 140,5:321; and 140,10:778)

Annals of Nutrition and Metabolism (47,6:306)

Archives of Dermatology (134,11:1349; 138,2:207; and 140,5:563)

Archives of Internal Medicine (160,21:3329; 162,12:1382; 162,18:2113; 163,12:1448; 163,13:1587; 164,11:1237; and 164,14:1534)

Archives of Neurology (57,6:831 and 57,10:1439)

Aromatherapy: A Lifetime Guide to Healing with Essential Oils, Prentice Hall, Englewood Cliffs, N.J., 1996

Arteriosclerosis, Thrombosis, and Vascular Biology (24,3:e25)

Arzneimittel-Forschung (49,11:900)

Atherosclerosis (148,1:49)

Athletic Therapy Today (9,5:52)

B

Bacteria For Breakfast, Trafford Publishing, Victoria, B.C., Canada, 2003

Baking Soda <www.armhammer.com> retrieved Feb. 21, 2005

Biofactors (18,1-4:153)

Bionic Foods, KATU <www.katu.com> retrieved Dec. 14, 2004

BMC Psychiatry (3,1:17)

Botanical Medicines: The desk reference for major herbal supplements, The Haworth Herbal Press, New York, 2002

Botox Cosmetic: A Look at Looking Good, U.S. Food and Drug Administration, FDA Consumer <www.fda.gov> retrieved Jan. 11, 2005

Botulinum Toxin A Improves Refractory Benign Prostatic Hyperplasia Symptoms: Paper presented at American Urological Association 2004 annual meeting; May 11, 2004; San Francisco, Calif.

Botulinum Toxin, American Academy of Dermatology <www.aad.org> retrieved Jan. 11, 2005

Brain Food: Puzzles for the brain to gnaw on, RinkWorks <www.RinkWorks.com/brainfood> retrieved Aug. 23, 2004

Brazilian Journal of Medical and Biological Research (36,10:1409 and 37,7:1029)

British Journal of Dermatology (147:1212)

British Journal of Medicine (327,7407:128)

British Medical Journal (322,7278:73; 323,7327:1446; 325,7376:1312; 327,7429:1454; 328,7446:991; and 328,7453:1395)

Bronchial asthma: The scale of the problem, World Health Organization <www.who.int> retrieved Jan. 4, 2005

C

CA A Cancer Journal for Clinicians (53,1:5)

Calcium, ConsumerLab.com <www.ConsumerLab.com> retrieved Jan. 6, 2005

Canadian Medical Association Journal (170,4:477)

Cancer (95,11:2390)

Cancer Causes and Control (14,1:1)

Cancer Epidemiology, Biomarkers & Prevention (12,7:597)

Cancer Research (63,18:6096 and 64,23:8485)

Cartilage (Bovine and Shark), National Cancer Institute, U.S. National Institutes of Health <www.cancer.gov> retrieved Jan. 20, 2005

Center for Science in the Public Interest news release, March 21, 2000

Chelation Therapy: Unproven Claims and Unsound Theories, Quackwatch <www.quackwatch.org> retrieved Aug. 19, 2004

Chest (122,5:1535 and 125,6:2011)

Chiropractic Quick Facts, International Chiropractors Association <www.chiropractic.org> retrieved on Dec. 28, 2004

Chitosan, ConsumerLab.com <www.consumerlab.com> retrieved Nov. 9, 2004

Chitosan: A Critical Look, Quackwatch <www.quackwatch.org> retrieved Aug. 19, 2004

Cholesterol Lowering Supplements (Guggulsterones, Policosanol, Sterols), ConsumerLab.com <www.consumerlab.com> retrieved Aug. 1, 2003

Christopher Gardner Ph.D., assistant professor, Department of Medicine, Stanford University, Stanford Calif.

Circulation (98,9:935; 106,21:2747; and 107,7:947)

Cleveland Clinic Journal of Medicine (71,4:327 and 71,9:746)

Clinical and Experimental Dermatology (28:232)

Clinical Infectious Diseases (35,12:1566 and 38,10:1367,1413)

Clinical Otolaryngology (29,3:226)

Clinical Trial: Nonpharmacologic Analgesia for Invasive Procedures, National Institutes of Health <www.clinicaltrials.gov> retrieved Jan. 24, 2005

Cochrane Database of Systematic Reviews (Online: Update Software) The Cochrane Database of Systematic Reviews 01-JAN-2002(3):CD003335

Cocoavia, Frequently Asked Questions, Mars Incorporated <www.cocoavia.com> retrieved Dec. 2, 2004

Coenzyme Q10, ConsumerLab <www.consumerlab.com> retrieved Jan. 13, 2004

Consumer Reports (68,7: 30; 69,8:45; and 69,5:12)

ConsumerLab.com news release (Dec. 22, 2003)

Cool Tips for Hot Gardeners, The Epsom Salt Industry Council <www.epsomsaltcouncil.org> retrieved July 24, 2003

Coronary Heart Disease: The Johns Hopkins White Papers, Medletter Associates, Inc., New York, 2004

Coverage Issues Manual Medical Procedures, Medicare <www.medicare.gov> retrieved Dec. 2, 2004

Critical Reviews in Food Science and Nutrition (43,1:1)

CSPI's Guide to Food Additives, Center for Science in the Public Interest <www.cspinet.org> retrieved Oct. 29, 2004

Current Atherosclerosis Reports (5,6:468)

Current Opinion in Clinical Nutrition and Metabolic Care (6,6:657)

Current Opinions in Lipidology (13,1:41)

Current Treatment Options in Gastroenterology (6,4:283)

Cutis (73,2:107)

D

Dana Carpender's Carb Gram Counter, Fair Winds Press, Gloucester, Mass., 2004

DeLee and Drez's Orthopaedic Sports Medicine, Elsevier, Philadelphia, 2004

Dementia and Geriatric Cognitive Disorders (17,3:109)

Depression and Anxiety (18,4:163)

Depression, NIH Publication No. 02-3561, National Institute of Mental Health, Bethesda, MD 20892

DHEA supplements, ConsumerLab <www.consumerlab.com> retrieved Dec. 11, 2002

Diabetes Care (26,4:1147; 26,7:2211; 26,12:3215; 27,1:134; and 27,8:2047)

Diabetes Mellitus, Integrative Medicine <www.onemedicine.com> retrieved Feb. 7, 2002

Diabetes Technology & Therapeutics (2,3:401)

Diabetic Medicine (16,12:1040)

Dietary Reference Intakes for Vitamin A, Vitamin K, Arsenic, Boron, Chromium, Copper, Iodine, Iron, Manganese, Molybdenum, Nickel, Silicon, Vanadium, and Zinc, National Academy Press, Washington, 2001

Dietary Supplement Fact Sheet: Calcium, Office of Dietary Supplements, National Institutes of Health <www.ods.od.nih.gov> retrieved Dec. 9, 2004

Dietary Supplement Fact Sheet: Vitamin B12, Office of Dietary Supplements, National Institutes of Health <www.ods.od.nih.gov> retrieved Dec. 28, 2004

Dietary Supplement Fact Sheet: Vitamin D, Office of Dietary Supplements, National Institutes of Health <www.ods.od.nih.gov> retrieved Dec. 10, 2004

Dietary Supplements, Pharmaceutical Press, London, 2001

Digestive and Liver Disease (34,1:29 and 34,1:22)

Digestive Diseases and Sciences (47,9:2079 and 49,7-8:1088)

Digestive Disorders: The Johns Hopkins White Papers, Medletter Associates, Inc., New York, 2004

Discopathy with leg pain: A randomized controlled trial of Orthotrac vs EZBRACE <www.spineuniverse.com> retrieved Jan. 10, 2005

Dr. Dean Ornish's Program for Reversing Heart Disease, Random House, New York, 1990

Drug Facts and Comparisons, Facts and Comparisons, Inc., St. Louis, Mo., 1995

Drug Information, PDRhealth <www.pdrhealth.com> retrieved Oct.18, 2004

Drug monograph: Ibuprofen, Clinical Pharmacology <www.ClinicalPharmacology.com> retrieved Sept. 17, 2004

Drugs (56,3:307; 57,6:855; and 63,9:845)

E

Effects of Omega-3 Fatty Acids on Lipids and Glycemic Control in Type II Diabetes and the Metabolic Syndrome and on Inflammatory Bowel Disease, Rheumatoid Arthritis, Renal Disease, Systemic Lupus Erythematosus, and Osteoporosis, Evidence Report/Technology Assessment No. 89, AHRQ Publication No. 04-E012-1, Agency for Healthcare Research and Quality, Rockville, MD 20850

Emergency Medicine (36,7:20)

Emotional Intelligence, Bantam Books, New York, 1995

Environmental Health Perspectives (108,5:435)

Environmental Nutrition, July 2003

European Journal of Clinical Nutrition (53,5:379; 56,9:830; 57,2:293; and 57,5:721)

European Journal of Dermatology (10,8:596)

European Journal of Gastroenterology and Hepatology (14,5:521)

European Respiratory Journal (15,6:996)

Experimental and Clinical Endocrinology & Diabetes (108,3:168)

F

Fact Sheet: Evaluating medical research findings and clinical trials, Family Caregiver Alliance <www.caregiver.org> retrieved Jan. 27, 2005

Fact Sheets: Osteoporosis Overview, National Institutes of Health Osteoporosis and Related Bone Diseases — National Resource Center <www.osteo.org> retrieved Dec. 3, 2004

FDA Consumer (28,10:15; 33,6:12; 35,1:12)

FDA Talk Paper: FDA Authorizes New Coronary Heart Disease Health Claim for Plant Sterol and Plant Stanol Esters, Food and Drug Administration <www.cfsan.fda.gov> retrieved Dec. 20, 2004

Federal Trade Commission news release (March 17, 2004)

Fertility and Sterility (80,6:1495)

Fish Oil Natural Remedy, McKesson Health Solutions, McKesson Corporation Headquarters, One Post Street, San Francisco, CA 94104-5296

Food Insight (July/August 2002)

Food Storage Guide: Answers the Question, North Dakota State University Extension Service <www.ext.nodak.edu> retrieved Dec. 30, 2004

Free Radical Biology & Medicine (27,3-4:309)

Free Radical Research (31,3:171)

From Test Tube to Patient: Improving health through human drugs, Publication No. 017-012-00400-8, Superintendent of Documents, P.O. Box 371954, Pittsburgh, PA 15250-7954

G

Garlic Supplements, ConsumerLab.com <www.consumerlab.com> retrieved Oct. 30, 2002

Garlic: Effects on Cardiovascular Risks and Disease, Protective Effects Against Cancer, and Clinical Adverse Effects. Summary, Evidence Report/Technology Assessment: Number 20. AHRQ Publication No. 01-E022, October 2000. Agency for Healthcare Research and Quality, Rockville, MD 20850

General Shelf Lives for Common Items, California State University Northridge <www.csun.edu> retrieved Dec. 30, 2004

Geriatrics (57,5:24; 58,2:28; and 58,3:30)

Gerontology (49:380)

Ginseng, ConsumerLab.com <www.consumerlab.com> retrieved Aug. 29, 2003

Gut (53,11:1617)

H

H. pylori and peptic ulcer, NIH Publication No. 01-4225, National Digestive Diseases Information Clearinghouse, 2 Information Way, Bethesda, MD 20892

Heart and Lung (32,6:368)

Heart Attack Prevention: The Johns Hopkins White Papers, Medletter Associates, Inc., New York, 2004

Home Remedies for Pest Control, U.S. Army Center for Health Promotion and Preventive Medicine <chppm-www.apgea.army.mil> Feb. 21, 2005

Home Remedies, Holistic Approach, Repellent Plants, The Ohio State University <http://ohioline.osu.edu> retrieved July 17, 2003

Hospital Practice (36,8:55)

Hot Tubs and High Blood Pressure, American Heart Association <www.americanheart.org> retrieved Sept. 1, 2004

How Blood Pressure Pill Prevents Heart Attacks, Rednova News <www.rednova.com> retrieved Aug. 31, 2004

How to help your Allergies and Asthma, The American Academy of Allergies, Asthma and Immunology, 555 E. Wells St., Ste. 1100, Milwaukee, Wisc.

How to Understand and Interpret Food and Health-Related Scientific Studies, International Food Information Council Foundation, 1100 Connecticut Ave., N.W., Suite 430, Washington, DC 20036

Hypertension and Stroke: The Johns Hopkins White Papers, Medletter Associates, Inc., New York, 2004

Hypertensive patients have increased sensitivity to meteorological parameters for myocardial infarction occurrence; Paper presented at: European Society of Cardiology Congress; 2004; Munich, Germany

Hypnotherapy, Hypnosis, Intelihealth.com
<www.intelihealth.com> retrieved Jan. 24, 2005

I

Ingvar Bjelland, M.D., Ph.D., University of Bergen,
Bergen, Norway

*International Journal of Clinical Pharmacology and
Therapeutics* (42,2:63)

International Journal of Cosmetic Science (26,3:169)

International Journal of Food Science and Nutrition
(55,3:223)

Interpreting News on Diet, Harvard School of Public Health
<www.hsph.harvard.edu> retrieved Jan. 17, 2005

Is antibacterial soap any better than regular soap?
Howstuffworks <http://home.howstuffworks.com>
retrieved Oct. 22, 2004

J

Jennifer Grana, registered dietician, Highmark, Inc.,
Pittsburgh, Penn.

Joanne Borg-Stein, M.D., chief of service of Physical
Medicine and Rehabilitation, Newton-Wellesley Hospital,
Newton, Mass.

John Robbins, M.D., professor of medicine, University of
California, Davis, Calif.

John W. Farquhar, M.D., professor of Medicine and
Health Research and Policy, Emeritus (Active), Stanford
Prevention Research Center, Stanford University School of
Medicine, Stanford, Calif.

Johns Hopkins Medical Letter Health After 50 (15,12:8)

Journal of Advanced Nursing (44,5:517)

Journal of Agricultural and Food Chemistry (49,3:1625
51,25:7292)

Journal of Allergy and Clinical Immunology (104,2Pt1:447
and 112,3:513)

Journal of Antimicrobial Chemotherapy (39,3:393)

Journal of Cardiovascular Pharmacology (34,5:690)

Journal of Clinical Endocrinology and Metabolism
(88,7:3190 and 88,12:6015)

Journal of Clinical Oncology (16,11:3649)

Journal of Dermatological Treatment (10,2:119)

Journal of Epidemiology and Community Health (57,11:907)

Journal of Family Practice (51,5:425; 52,6:468; and
52,10:766)

Journal of Food Science (69,9:S357)

Journal of Hypertension (18,4:411)

Journal of Internal Medicine (255,1:89)

Journal of Manipulative and Physiological Therapeutics (26,5:e15)

Journal of Medicinal Food (6,2:79,87)

Journal of Neurology, Neurosurgery, and Psychiatry (75,8:1093)

Journal of Nutrition (127,4:579; 130,2S:268S; 133,4:1060; 133,9:2879; 134,3:562; 134,4:919; and 134,12:3412S)

Journal of Pain and Symptom Management (26,2:731)

Journal of Strength and Conditioning Research (16,3:416; 17,3:475; and 18,3:522)

Journal of the American Academy of Dermatology (50,4:541)

Journal of the American College of Cardiology (41,3:420 and 41,6:961)

Journal of the American College of Nutrition (19,5:578 and 20,5Suppl:363S; 22,4:283; 22,5:372; 22,6:519,533; and 23,3:197)

Journal of the American Dietetic Association (101,9:1006; 103,2:215; 103,10:1319; 104,2:255; and 104,5:814)

Journal of the American Geriatrics Society 52,4:540

Journal of the American Medical Association (280,17:1518; 287,14:1807; 287,23:3082; 288,7:835; 289,21:2819; 289,22:2947; 290,6:765; 290,8:1029; 290,17:2292; 291,10:1199,1213; 291,20:2433; 292,7:828; and 292,16:1955)

Journal of the American Nutraceutical Association (3,4:24)

Journal of the European Academy of Dermatology and Venereology (14,4:251)

Journal of the National Cancer Institute (95,21:1561)

Joye Willcox, Ph.D, registered dietician, owner of Healthy Diets, Inc., Raleigh, N.C.

L

Lippincott's Primary Care Practice (3,3:291)

Lona Sandon, R.D., M.Ed., assistant professor of clinical nutrition, The University of Texas Southwestern Medical Center at Dallas, Texas

Lutein and Zeaxanthin, ConsumerLab.com <www.consumerlab.com> retrieved Feb. 3, 2004

M

Maggie B. Covington, M.D., clinical sssistant professor of Family Medicine, University of Maryland, Baltimore, Md.

Magnesium, ConsumerLab <www.consumerlab.com> retrieved Jan. 7, 2005

Making Sense of Scientific Studies: Questions to Ask, American Cancer Society <www.cancer.org> retrieved Jan. 27, 2005

Mary B. Engler, Ph.D., professor and vascular physiologist, School of Nursing, University of California at San Francisco, San Francisco

Mary Beth Horrell, M.S., R.D., C.D.E., L.D.N., Diabetes and Health Education Center, Mission Hospital, Asheville, N.C.

Mayo Clinic Proceedings (76,12:1225; 77,11:1164; and 78,8:965)

Medical Encyclopedia: Essential tremor, MedlinePlus <www.nlm.nih.gov/medlineplus> retrieved Aug. 20, 2004

Medical Science Monitor (9,2:CR84; 10,6:HY27; and 10,8:RA187)

Melatonin supplements, ConsumerLab.com <www.consumerlab.com> retrieved Jan. 12, 2005

Memory: The Johns Hopkins White Papers, Medletter Associates, Inc., New York 2004

Mercury Levels in Commercial Fish and Shellfish, U.S. Food and Drug Administration <www.cfsan.fda.gov> retrieved Dec. 14, 2004

Michael Seidman, M.D., director of the Otologic/Neurotologic Surgery Division, medical director for the Center for Integrative Medicine, Henry Ford Health Systems, West Bloomfield, Mich.

Michael Yelland, senior lecturer in general practice, University of Queensland, Australia

Mindi Miller, Pharm.D., BCPS (Board Certified Pharmacotherapy Specialist), clinical pharmacist, Emory Healthcare, Atlanta

Minnesota Medicine (85,11:42)

Miracle Health Claims: Add a dose of skepticism, Federal Trade Commission <www.ftc.gov> retrieved Nov. 11, 2004

Morbidity and Mortality Weekly Report (51,47:1065)

N

Nasal Strips: A Popular Snoring Cure, Here Be Dreams <www.here-be-dreams.com> retrieved Dec. 30, 2004

National Cancer Institute news release (April 25, 2002)

National Center for Health Statistics news release (Oct. 27, 2004)

National Institutes of Health news release (Sept. 30, 1999)

National Institutes of Health/National Heart, Lung, and Blood Institute news release (May 14, 2003)

Natural Products Encyclopedia: Zinc, ConsumerLab.com <www.consumerlab.com> retrieved Oct. 24, 2004

Nature (424,6952:1013 and 426,6968:787)

Nature Reviews Neuroscience (3,11:862)

Neuroepidemiology (23,1-2:94)

Neurology (60,9:1424,1429; 60,9:1429; 61,6:812; 61,9:1273; and 63,4:757)

New England Journal of Medicine (348,14:1322; 348,25:2489,2508; 350,20:2033,2042; and 351,4:315)

Nutrients in 100 grams of peanuts and tree nuts,
International Tree Nut Council <www.nuthealth.org>
retrieved Aug. 12, 2004

Nutrition & the M.D. (30,3:1)

*Nutrition Bars (Energy Bars, Protein Bars, Diet Bars, and
Meal-Replacement Bars),* ConsumerLab.com
<www.consumerlab.com> retrieved Feb. 7, 2005

Nutrition Concepts and Controversies,
Wadsworth/Thompson Learning, Belmont, Calif., 2000

Nutrition in Clinical Care (4,3:140)

Nutrition Journal (2,1:20)

Nutrition Reviews (62,1:18; 62,3:115; and 62,4:125)

Nutrition Today (37,3:103)

O

Obesity Research (11,5:683)

*Omega-3 Fatty Acids (EPA and DHA) from Fish/Marine
Oils,* ConsumerLab.com <www.ConsumerLab.com>
retrieved Oct. 7, 2004

Optometry (75,4:216)

Oral Hyaluronic Acid Knee Arthritis Study
<www.drreevesonline.com> retrieved Jan. 19, 2005

Orolaryngology Clinics of North America (36,2:359)

Osteoporosis Overview, National Institutes of Health <www.osteo.org> retrieved Dec. 3, 2004

Otolaryngology Clinics of North America (36,2:359)

Outcomes Management (6,3:132)

P

Pain (106,1-2:59)

Parkinson's Disease Foundation <www.pdf.org> retrieved Jan. 20, 2005

Parkinsonism and Related Disorders (8,5:343 and 9,6:341)

Paul Terry, Ph.D., assistant professor of Epidemiology, Emory University, Atlanta

Pediatric Emergency Care (19,3:169)

Penny Kris-Etherton, Ph.D., distinguished professor of Nutrition, Pennsylvania State University, University Park, Pa.

Peripheral Arterial Occlusive Disease: An Overview, eMedicine <www.emedicine.com> retrieved Nov. 3, 2004

Pharmacological Research (48,5:511)

Pharmacotherapy (23,7:871)

Philippe Szapary, assistant professor of medicine, University of Pennsylvania School of Medicine, Philadelphia

Physiological Research (52,4:397)

Phytomedicine (9,1:3)

Pizzorno: Textbook of Natural Medicine, Churchill Livingstone, Inc., New York, 1999

Plasma Lycopene and the Risk of Cardiovascular Disease in Women, Paper presented at: American College of Cardiology 2002 annual meeting March 2002; Atlanta

Plastic and Reconstructive Surgery (104,4:1110)

Platelets (14,5:325)

Probiotic Supplements and Foods (Including Lactobacillus acidophilus and Bifidobacterium), Consumerlab <www.consumerlab.com> retrieved Jan. 7, 2005

Proceedings of the National Academy of Sciences of the United States of America (99,11:7610; 100,7:3766; and 101,9:3316)

Prolo your back pain away, Beulah Land Press, Oak Park, Ill., 2000

Promoting a Physically Active Lifestyle through Alternative Forms of Exercise, Paper presented at the American College of Sports Medicine's 2004 conference; University of Pittsburgh, Pittsburgh, Pa.

Prostate Disorders: The Johns Hopkins White Papers, Medletter Associates, Inc., New York, 2004

Psychosomatic Medicine (66,4:599)

Psychotherapy and Psychosomatics (72,2:59,80)

Q

Qualified Health Claims: Letter of Enforcement Discretion — Nuts and Coronary Heart Disease, Food and Drug Administration <www.cfsan.fda.gov> retrieved Jan. 13, 2005

Questions & Answers: Flu Vaccine, Centers for Disease Control and Prevention <www.cdc.gov> retrieved Jan. 21, 2005

Questions and Answers, Qualified Health Claim for Omega-3 Fatty Acids, Eicosapentaenoic Acid (EPA) and Docosahexaenoic Acid (DHA), U.S. Food and Drug Administration <www.cfsan.fda.gov> retrieved Oct. 10, 2004

R

Residential Air Cleaning Devices: A Summary of Available Information, Indoor Air Publications <www.epa.gov> retrieved Jan. 12, 2005

Review of Medical Physiology, Appleton & Lange, Stamford, Conn., 1999

RN (64,1:42)

Robert P. Heaney, M.D., professor of medicine, Creighton University, Omaha, Neb.

Ryan J. Huxtable, professor emeritus, University of Arizona, Tucson, Ariz.

S

Saint Louis University Health Sciences Center press release (March 29, 2004)

Sally Stabler, M.D, professor of medicine and co-head of the hematology division, University of Colorado Health Sciences Center, Denver

SAMe, Consumer Lab <www.ConsumerLab.com> retrieved Oct. 20, 2004

Saturday Evening Post (March/April 2004)

Saw Palmetto, ConsumerLab.com <www.consumerlab.com> retrieved May 21, 2003

Science (286,5444:1558 and 303,5655:226)

Science News (140,2:20)

Sharon Alger-Mayer, physician-nutrition specialist and associate professor of medicine, Albany Medical College, Albany, N.Y.

Sinusitis, Health Matters, National Institute of Allergy and Infectious Diseases <www.niaid.nih.gov> retrieved Feb. 17, 2005

Snoring, TipsOfAllSorts.com <www.tipsofallsorts.com> retrieved Dec. 30, 2004

Spine (27,20:2193 and 29,1:9)

Spirulina, Green Superfood For Life <www.spirulina.com> retrieved Jan. 31, 2005

St. John's Wort and the Treatment of Depression, National Center for Complementary and Alternative Medicine, <www.nccam.nih.gov> retrieved Jan. 19, 2003

St. John's Wort, ConsumerLab.com <www.consumerlab.com> retrieved May 3, 2004

Statins, National Heart Lung and Blood Institute <http://nhlbisupport.com> retrieved Nov. 11, 2004

Stevia: The Genus Stevia, Taylor & Francis, New York, 2002

Stroke (31,10:2287)

Support Care Cancer (11,4:232)

Swiss Medical Weekly (132,25-26:338)

T

Technology Assessment: Acupuncture for Osteoarthritis, U.S. Department of Health and Human Services, Public Health Service, The Agency for Healthcare Research and Quality, 540 Gaither Road, Rockville, MD 20850

Textbook of Family Practice, W.B. Saunders Company, Philadelphia, 2000

Textbook of Natural Medicine, Churchill Livingstone, Inc., Kenmore, Wash., 1999

The 2004 Surgeon General's Report on Bone Health and Osteoporosis: What It Means To You, U.S. Department of Health and Human Services, Office of the Surgeon General, 2004

The Arthritis Cure, St. Martin's Griffin, New York, 2004

The Arthritis Foundation <www.arthritis.org> retrieved Oct. 21, 2004

The Arthritis Foundation's Guide to Alternative Therapies, Arthritis Foundation, Atlanta, 1999

The Common Cold, National Institute of Allergy and Infectious Diseases, National Institutes of Health <www.niaid.nih.gov> retrieved Jan. 19, 2005

The Effect of Ready to Eat Cereal consumption on Macronutrient Intakes and Body Mass Index (BMI) in American adults, Paper presented at: Experimental Biology 2003 meeting; April 11-15, 2003; San Diego, Calif.

The International Essential Tremor Foundation <www.essentialtremor.org> retrieved Jan. 5, 2005

The Journal for Urology (172,1:20)

The Journal of Clinical Endocrinology & Metabolism (89,3:1217)

The Journal of Family Practice (52,6:468)

The Journal of Neuroscience (23,12:5088)

The Journal of Nutrition (133,3:801)

The Journal of Nutrition, Health & Aging (8,2:92)

The Lancet (355,9214:1486; 357,9249:4; 361,9357:543; 361,9368:1491,1496; 362,9400:2012; 363,9415:1139; and 364,9437:897)

The New Yoga, YogaJournal.com <www.yogajournal.com> retrieved Jan. 20, 2005

The Physician and Sports Medicine (32,7:41)

The Review of Natural Products, Facts and Comparisons Publishing Group, St. Louis, Mo., 2004

The Seventh Annual Report of the Joint National Committee on the Prevention, Detection, Evaluation, and Treatment of High Blood Pressure, NIH Publication No. 04-5230, U.S. Department of Health and Human Services; National Institutes of Health; National Heart, Lung, and Blood Institute; National High Blood Pressure Education Program; August 2004

The Use of Complementary and Alternative Medicine in the United States: CAM Therapies Used the Most, National Center for Complementary and Alternative Medicine <http://nccam.nih.gov> retrieved Sept. 1, 2004

The Wall Street Journal (Dec. 23, 2003, D5; March 17, 2004, D1; and Oct. 7, 2003, D1)

The Wall Street Journal Online <http://online.wsj.com> (Nov. 19, 2002; Dec. 30, 2003; Jan. 27, 2004; and July 22, 2003)

Thorax (57,2:110)

Timothy Roehrs, Ph.D., director of research, Sleep Disorders and Research Center, Henry Ford Hospital, Detroit

U

U.S. Food and Drug Administration news release (Feb. 6, 2004)

U.S. Pharmacist (29,5:16)

U.S. Senate Committee on Appropriations news release (July 15, 2004)

Understanding NSAID-induced ulcers, Elfstrom <http://elfstrom.com/arthritis/nsaids> retrieved Sept. 16, 2004

University of California Berkeley Wellness Letter, May 2003

Urology (62,2:259)

W

Weight Loss, Slimming, and Diabetes-Management Supplements (Chromium, CLA, and Pyruvate), ConsumerLab.com <www.consumerlab.com> retrieved Aug. 27, 2004

Welcome to All-Star Puzzles, All-Star Puzzles <www.AllStarPuzzles.com> retrieved Aug. 23, 2004

Western Journal of Medicine (171,3:168 and 175,4:269)

What Causes High Blood Pressure? National Heart, Lung, and Blood Institute <www.nhlbi.nih.gov> retrieved Sept. 1, 2004

What is stress? A.D.A.M., Inc. 1600 River Edge Parkway, Suite 100, Atlanta, GA 30328

What to do for colds and flu, (FDA) 00-1280, Department of Health and Human Services, Food and Drug Administration, 5600 Fishers Lane (HFI-40), Rockville, MD 20857

What You Need to Know About Mercury in Fish and Shellfish, Food and Drug Administration <www.cfsan.fda.gov> retrieved Oct. 20, 2004

Why Is High Blood Pressure Important? National Heart, Lung, and Blood Institute <www.nhlbi.nih.gov> retrieved Sept. 1, 2004

Wrigley <www.wrigley.com> retrieved Jan. 11, 2005

Y

Your guide to lowering high blood pressure, National Heart, Lung, and Blood Institute <www.nhlbi.nih.gov> retrieved Sept. 10, 2004

Index